PharmacologyPro

Gerard Browne

PharmacologyPro

A Practical Guide for Anaesthesiology Exams

Springer

Gerard Browne
Department of Anaesthesiology
Tallaght University Hospital
Dublin, Ireland

ISBN 978-3-032-10226-3 ISBN 978-3-032-10227-0 (eBook)
https://doi.org/10.1007/978-3-032-10227-0

This Springer imprint is published by the registered company Springer Nature Switzerland AG
The registered company address is: Gewerbestrasse 11, 6330 Cham, Switzerland

Acknowledgements

The author would like to thank the anaesthesia trainees whose questions, feedback, and enthusiasm inspired the structure and scope of this book. A most sincere thank you to Adrian and Bernie, without their support, this could not have been possible.

Declaration of Competing Interests The author declares no competing financial interests or personal relationships that could have influenced the content of this textbook.

Disclaimer: Dosages used in this book are for educational purposes. Clinical decisions and dosages should be based on a local formulary and local guidelines.

About the Book

PharmacologyPro: A Practical Guide for Anaesthesiology Exams is a comprehensive reference designed to support anaesthesiologists, intensivists, and trainees preparing for postgraduate examinations such as the FRCA, FCAI, EDAIC, and FANZCA. Written with a practical clinical focus, the book bridges the gap between pharmacological theory and its direct application in perioperative and critical care practice.

Organised by drug class, each chapter provides a structured overview of key agents including their mechanism of action, pharmacokinetics, clinical uses, adverse effects, and dosing considerations. Special attention is given to anaesthesia-specific drugs such as intravenous anaesthetic agents, neuromuscular blockers, local anaesthetics, opioids, and adjuvant medications, alongside critical care agents such as vasoactive drugs, anticoagulants, and antimicrobials.

The book is structured to facilitate both rapid revision and in-depth study. Didactic elements such as tables, key point summaries, and comparative drug charts enhance readability and provide quick reference for clinicians in training and practice. References at the end of each chapter guide the reader towards further study and evidence-based sources.

This text will be of value to anaesthesiology trainees at all stages, consultant anaesthesiologists seeking a concise pharmacology reference, and allied health professionals working in operating theatres, recovery units, and intensive care settings.

Contents

1 Fundamentals of Pharmacology 1
- 1.1 Drug Action 1
- 1.2 Receptors 3
- 1.3 Enzyme Inducers & Inhibitors 6
- 1.4 First and Zero Order Kinetics 8
- 1.5 Isomers 9
- 1.6 Summary 10
- References 11

2 Pharmacokinetics 13
- 2.1 Absorption and Bioavailability 13
- 2.2 Drug Metabolism 15
- 2.3 Half Life and Clearance 17
- 2.4 Compartment Models 18
- References 20

3 Cardiac Drugs 23
- 3.1 Anti-Arrhythmic Drugs 23
- 3.2 Antihypertensive Drugs 32
- 3.3 Vasopressors & Inotropes 47
- References 56

4 Analgesics 61
- 4.1 NSAIDS 61
- 4.2 Opioids 67
- References 76

5 Antiemetic Drugs 79
- 5.1 Antiemetic Drugs 79
- 5.2 Domperidone 81
- 5.3 Prochlorperazine 82
- 5.4 Metoclopramide 83
- 5.5 Cyclizine 84
- 5.6 Ondansetron 85
- 5.7 Dexamethasone 86
- 5.8 Aprepitant 88
- References 89

6 Central Nervous System Drugs . . . 91
6.1 Anticonvulsant Drugs . . . 91
6.2 Antidepressant Drugs . . . 99
6.3 Hypnotic Drugs . . . 108
References . . . 112

7 Anti-Diabetic Medication . . . 115
7.1 Anti-Diabetic Drugs . . . 115
7.2 Biguanides . . . 117
7.3 Sulphonylureas . . . 118
7.4 SGLT2 Inhibitors . . . 119
7.5 GLP-1 Mimetics . . . 120
7.6 DPP4 Inhibitors . . . 122
7.7 Alpha-Glucosidase Inhibitors . . . 123
7.8 Thiazolidinediones . . . 124
7.9 Insulin . . . 126
References . . . 128

8 Diuretics . . . 131
8.1 Diuretic Drugs . . . 131
8.2 Furosemide . . . 132
8.3 Thiazide Diuretics . . . 133
8.4 Mannitol . . . 135
8.5 Amiloride . . . 136
8.6 Spironolactone . . . 137
8.7 Acetozolamide . . . 138
References . . . 140

9 Drugs Acting on Blood . . . 143
9.1 Blood Products . . . 143
9.2 Anticoagulant Drugs . . . 151
9.3 Antiplatelet Drugs . . . 159
References . . . 168

10 Anaesthesiology Drugs . . . 173
10.1 Intravenous Anaesthetic Agents . . . 173
10.2 Inhalational Anaesthetic Agents . . . 183
10.3 Neuromuscular Blocking Drugs . . . 187
10.4 Local Anaesthetics . . . 193
References . . . 199

11 Questions on Pharmacology Fundamentals . . . 203

12 Questions on Clinical Drugs . . . 209

Index . . . 221

About the Author

Gerard Browne is a Consultant Anaesthesiologist at Tallaght University Hospital in Dublin, with a special interest in regional anaesthesia, trauma anaesthesia, and pharmacology. He completed his specialist training through the College of Anaesthesiologists of Ireland and has held fellowship positions in trauma, regional and obstetric anaesthesia. He is passionate about structured education and has developed simulation bootcamps and examination-focused curricula for anaesthesia trainees. This textbook stems from years of experience teaching pharmacology to candidates preparing for national and international postgraduate anaesthesia examinations.

Abbreviations

ACE	Angiotensin-Converting Enzyme
ACh	Acetylcholine
ADR	Adverse Drug Reaction
AF	Atrial Fibrillation
AV	Atrioventricular
BBB	Blood-Brain Barrier
BP	Blood Pressure
CINV	Chemotherapy-Induced Nausea and Vomiting
CNS	Central Nervous System
CO	Cardiac Output
COX	Cyclooxygenase
CRP	C-Reactive Protein
CTZ	Chemoreceptor Trigger Zone
CYP	Cytochrome P450 Enzyme System
DVT	Deep Vein Thrombosis
ECG	Electrocardiogram
ED50	Effective Dose for 50% of Population
EMLA	Eutectic Mixture of Local Anaesthetics
FFP	Fresh Frozen Plasma
GABA	Gamma-Aminobutyric Acid
GFR	Glomerular Filtration Rate
GLP	Glucagon-Like Peptide
GPCR	G-Protein Coupled Receptor
GTN	Glyceryl Trinitrate
HIT	Heparin-Induced Thrombocytopenia
HR	Heart Rate
ICP	Intracranial Pressure
ICU	Intensive Care Unit
IM	Intramuscular
INR	International Normalised Ratio
IV	Intravenous
LA	Local Anaesthetic
LAST	Local Anaesthetic Systemic Toxicity
MAC	Minimum Alveolar Concentration

MAO	Monoamine Oxidase
MAP	Mean Arterial Pressure
MI	Myocardial Infarction
N+V	Nausea and Vomiting
NMBA	Neuromuscular Blocking Agent
NMDA	N-Methyl-D-Aspartate
NSAID	Non-Steroidal Anti-Inflammatory Drug
P450	Cytochrome P450 Enzyme
PCC	Prothrombin Complex Concentrate
PE	Pulmonary Embolism
PONV	Post-Operative Nausea and Vomiting
RAAS	Renin-Angiotensin-Aldosterone System
SC	Subcutaneous
SGLT	Sodium-Glucose Co-Transporter
SSRI	Selective Serotonin Reuptake Inhibitor
SVR	Systemic Vascular Resistance
TCI	Target-Controlled Infusion
TIVA	Total Intravenous Anaesthesia
TOF	Train-of-Four
TPMT	Thiopurine Methyltransferase
TRALI	Transfusion-Related Acute Lung Injury
Vd	Volume of Distribution

Fundamentals of Pharmacology

1

1.1 Drug Action

Mechanisms of Drug Action

Drugs exert their effects through several key mechanisms. Receptors are proteins that bind ligands such as hormones or neurotransmitters to initiate intracellular signalling cascades; these are discussed in greater detail in the next chapter (Brunton 2018a, b). Ion channels may be blocked or modulated by drugs—for instance, local anaesthetics inhibit voltage-gated sodium channels to prevent nerve conduction (Rang and Henderson 2016). Enzymes can be inhibited or activated, as seen with ibuprofen, which blocks cyclooxygenase (COX) enzymes to reduce prostaglandin synthesis (Vanderah 2021). Hormone production may be altered pharmacologically; for example, carbimazole inhibits the synthesis of thyroid hormones. Neurotransmitter activity is commonly modified by drugs that inhibit reuptake or breakdown, such as selective serotonin reuptake inhibitors (SSRIs), which increase synaptic serotonin levels. Transport systems across cell membranes may also be targeted, as demonstrated by digoxin's inhibition of the Na^+/K^+-ATPase pump (Vanderah 2021). Lastly, some drugs exert physicochemical actions through direct chemical interaction—for example, antacids neutralise gastric hydrochloric acid.

Receptor Binding Terms

1. Agonist: A drug that binds to a receptor and produces a biological response.
   Example: Morphine is a full agonist at the μ-opioid receptor.
2. Antagonist: A drug that binds to a receptor but does not activate it; it blocks or dampens the effect of agonists. Two key types:
   1. Competitive (Reversible) Antagonist:
      Binds reversibly; effect can be overcome by increasing agonist concentration.
      Example: Naloxone at opioid receptors.

G. Browne, *PharmacologyPro*, https://doi.org/10.1007/978-3-032-10227-0_1

2. Non-Competitive (Irreversible) Antagonist:
   Either binds irreversibly or causes a conformational change in the receptor that prevents agonist activation.
   Example: Ketamine at the NMDA receptor.
3. Partial Agonist: Binds to the receptor but produces only a partial response, even at full receptor occupancy.
   Example: Buprenorphine at opioid receptors.
4. Inverse Agonist: Binds to the same receptor as an agonist but induces the opposite response (i.e. suppresses baseline activity of constitutively active receptors).
   Example: Antihistamines at H_1 receptors.

Drug Potency
Potency describes the amount of drug required to produce a specific pharmacological effect. A highly potent drug achieves its desired effect at a low concentration, whereas a drug of low potency requires a much higher dose to produce the same response. Potency is typically quantified using the EC_{50}, which is the concentration of drug that produces 50% of its maximal effect (Kenakin 2014). For example, fentanyl is more potent than morphine because it produces equivalent analgesia at a much lower dose, while midazolam is more potent than diazepam as a sedative–hypnotic (Katzung and Vanderah 2021). Understanding drug potency is important when selecting agents and determining appropriate dosing regimens in clinical practice.

Therapeutic Index
The therapeutic index (TI) is a measure of drug safety, defined as the ratio of the median toxic dose (TD_{50}) to the median effective dose (ED_{50}) (Brunton 2018a, b). A high therapeutic index indicates a wide safety margin, meaning that toxic effects occur only at doses much higher than those required for efficacy. For example, paracetamol has a relatively high TI under normal conditions, making it generally safe at therapeutic doses. In contrast, a low therapeutic index reflects a narrow margin between effective and toxic doses, as seen with drugs such as digoxin and warfarin, which require careful monitoring to avoid potentially serious adverse effects (Calabrese and Baldwin 2003).

Types of Drug Interactions
Drug interactions can be classified as physicochemical, pharmacokinetic, or pharmacodynamic (Stockley 2010). Physicochemical interactions occur outside the body, such as in intravenous lines or in the gastrointestinal tract, due to physical or chemical incompatibility. An example is the precipitation of calcium and phosphate when mixed in solution. Pharmacokinetic interactions arise when one drug alters the absorption, distribution, metabolism, or excretion of another. For example, rifampicin, an enzyme inducer, reduces the plasma levels of many drugs by increasing their metabolism (Lin and Lu 1998). Pharmacodynamic interactions occur when

Table 1.1 Receptor types and drug examples

Receptor type	Example drugs	Clinical relevance
G Protein-Coupled Receptors (GPCRs)	Morphine (μ-opioid), Salbutamol (β2-agonist), Atropine (muscarinic antagonist)	Most common receptor type; site of action for many anaesthetic and cardiovascular drugs
Ligand-Gated Ion Channels	Benzodiazepines (GABA-A), Nicotine (nicotinic ACh), Ketamine (NMDA antagonist)	Rapid synaptic transmission; relevant in anaesthesia, epilepsy, muscle relaxants
Enzyme-Linked Receptors	Insulin, Trastuzumab (HER2 inhibitor)	Targeted in oncology and metabolic disease
Nuclear (Intracellular) Receptors	Steroids (e.g. dexamethasone), Thyroxine, Oestrogen	Important in endocrine modulation and long-term gene expression
Tyrosine Kinase Receptors	Insulin, Erlotinib (EGFR inhibitor)	Target for biologics and cancer therapeutics
Voltage-Gated Ion Channels	Lidocaine (Na+ blocker), Verapamil (Ca2+ blocker)	Key in anaesthesia and pain management

one drug modifies the effect of another at its site of action (Levy et al. 2000). These can include:

- **Summation (additive)**—the combined effect equals the sum of the individual effects (e.g., midazolam and fentanyl).
- **Synergism**—the combined effect exceeds the sum of the individual effects (e.g., propofol and alfentanil).
- **Potentiation**—a drug with no effect on its own enhances the effect of another (e.g., clavulanic acid enhances amoxicillin).
- **Antagonism**—one drug reduces or blocks the effect of another (e.g., naloxone antagonises morphine) (Table 1.1).

1.2 Receptors

Overview

Receptors are protein molecules, usually embedded within cell membranes, that mediate the actions of ligands such as drugs, neurotransmitters, or hormones (Hilal-Dandan and Brunton 2018). These receptors possess ligand-specific binding sites and are central to the pharmacodynamic effects of many therapeutic agents. A ligand is any molecule that binds to a receptor and may activate it, acting as an agonist, or block its activation, acting as an antagonist. The strength of the interaction between a ligand and its receptor is termed affinity, which influences how effectively the ligand can occupy the receptor (Neubig et al. 2003). The overall response to ligand binding depends on the receptor type, its anatomical location, and the downstream signalling pathways it modulates (Table 1.2).

The nicotinic acetylcholine (nACh) receptor is a well-characterised example of a ligand-gated ion channel. It is composed of five subunits arranged to form a central

Table 1.2 Classes of receptors

Receptor class	Location	Mechanism of action	Speed of response	Examples
Ligand-Gated Ion Channels	Cell membrane	Ligand binding opens an ion channel directly, allowing ion flow (Na^+, K^+, Cl^-, Ca^{2+}) across the membrane	Milliseconds	Nicotinic acetylcholine receptor (nAChR)
G Protein-Coupled Receptors (GPCRs)	Cell membrane	Ligand binding triggers a conformational change → activates G proteins (Gs, Gi, Gq) → modulates second messengers (e.g. cAMP, IP_3)	Seconds	Muscarinic ACh receptors, Adrenergic receptors, GABA-B
Receptor Tyrosine Kinases (RTKs)	Cell membrane (single-pass)	Ligand binding causes receptor dimerisation and autophosphorylation of tyrosine residues → activates intracellular kinase cascades	Minutes	Insulin receptor
Intracellular (Nuclear) Receptors	Cytoplasm or nucleus	Lipophilic ligand crosses membrane → binds intracellular receptor → ligand-receptor complex binds DNA → alters gene transcription	Hours	Glucocorticoid, thyroid hormone, oestrogen receptors

pore, specifically two α subunits, one β, one δ, and one γ subunit. Acetylcholine binds at the interface between the α and γ subunits, inducing a conformational change in the receptor structure. This change opens the central ion channel, allowing sodium ions (Na^+) to flow into the cell, which depolarises the cell membrane and initiates downstream signalling (Unwin 2005; Changeux 2012) (Table 1.3).

The second messengers cyclic AMP (cAMP) and cyclic GMP (cGMP) exert their effects through activation of protein kinases, specifically protein kinase A (PKA) and protein kinase G (PKG), respectively (Sutherland 1972). Inositol trisphosphate (IP_3) increases intracellular calcium levels by promoting calcium release from the endoplasmic reticulum, while diacylglycerol (DAG) activates protein kinase C (PKC), contributing to downstream signalling cascades (Hilal-Dandan and Brunton 2018).

Receptor Regulation and Tachyphylaxis

Receptor regulation describes changes in receptor number or sensitivity in response to chronic stimulation. Up-regulation refers to an increased number of receptors due to chronic under-stimulation; for example, patients with spinal cord injury may show heightened sensitivity to catecholamines (Insel 1996). In contrast, down-regulation occurs when chronic overstimulation decreases receptor number, as seen

Table 1.3 Second messengers in GPCR signalling

G protein type	Second messenger	Example receptors
Gs	↑ cAMP	β_1, β_2 adrenoceptors (e.g. salbutamol)
Gi	↓ cAMP	α_2 adrenoceptors, $\square_2$ mAChRs
Gq	↑ IP_3, ↑ DAG, ↑ Ca^{2+}	α_1 adrenoceptors, $\square_3$ mAChRs
–	↑ cGMP	Nitric oxide via guanylate cyclase activation

in insulin resistance associated with obesity (Lefkowitz 1998). Tachyphylaxis describes the rapid desensitisation to a drug after repeated dosing. Proposed mechanisms include receptor internalisation and depletion of intracellular mediators. A clinical example is the diminished pressor response to ephedrine when administered repeatedly during anaesthesia (Daly 2000).

NMDA Receptors
N-Methyl-D-Aspartate (NMDA) receptors are ligand-gated ion channels located in the central nervous system and are activated by glutamate, the brain's primary excitatory neurotransmitter (Collingridge et al. 2009). When stimulated, NMDA receptors allow the influx of sodium (Na^+) and calcium (Ca^{2+}) ions into neurons, playing a crucial role in synaptic plasticity, long-term potentiation, and central sensitisation. These mechanisms are fundamental to processes such as pain transmission, memory formation, and learning. Clinically, NMDA receptors serve as important drug targets; ketamine acts as a non-competitive NMDA antagonist, producing analgesic and dissociative anaesthesia, while nitrous oxide also exerts its effects in part through NMDA receptor antagonism (Petrenko et al. 2014).

GABA Receptors
Gamma-aminobutyric acid (GABA) is the principal inhibitory neurotransmitter in the central nervous system (CNS). It exerts its effects primarily through two receptor subtypes: GABA-A and GABA-B receptors. GABA-A receptors are ligand-gated chloride (Cl^-) channels composed of a pentameric structure typically consisting of two α, two β, and one γ or δ subunit. When GABA binds to these receptors, it facilitates the influx of Cl^- ions into the neuron, causing hyperpolarisation and thus neuronal inhibition. These receptors are the site of action for several anaesthetic and sedative agents, including benzodiazepines (which enhance the effect of GABA), as well as propofol, etomidate, and barbiturates (Olsen and Sieghart 2009). In contrast, GABA-B receptors are G-protein coupled receptors (GPCRs) that mediate inhibition through a different mechanism: they inhibit presynaptic calcium (Ca^{2+}) channels and activate postsynaptic potassium (K^+) channels, leading to reduced neuronal excitability. Baclofen is a commonly used drug that acts as a GABA-B receptor agonist (Bettler et al. 2004).

1.3 Enzyme Inducers & Inhibitors

Overview

The cytochrome P450 (CYP450) enzyme family plays a crucial role in the metabolism of more than 75% of drugs used in clinical practice. These enzymes are predominantly found in the liver but are also active in the intestines, lungs, and kidneys. Among the various CYP450 isoenzymes, two stand out for their clinical significance: CYP3A4, which is responsible for metabolising over half of all commonly prescribed medications, and CYP2D6, which is essential for the metabolism of many opioids, antidepressants, and beta-blockers (Zanger and Schwab 2013). The activity of CYP450 enzymes can be altered by drugs that act as inhibitors or inducers, leading to important pharmacokinetic interactions that may result in drug toxicity or therapeutic failure (Lin and Lu 2001).

Clinical Relevance

Alterations in drug metabolism due to enzyme inhibition or induction have important clinical implications. Enzyme inhibitors slow the metabolism of susceptible drugs, leading to increased plasma concentrations and a heightened risk of toxicity. Conversely, enzyme inducers accelerate metabolism, potentially lowering plasma drug levels and resulting in treatment failure. Drugs most at risk of significant interactions include those with a narrow therapeutic index, such as warfarin, phenytoin, theophylline, and ciclosporin (Wilkinson 2005). Additionally, drugs that are metabolised primarily by a single cytochrome P450 isoenzyme, or those that are highly protein-bound and exhibit high hepatic extraction ratios, are particularly vulnerable to clinically meaningful changes in pharmacokinetics (Pelkonen et al. 2008).

CYP450 Enzyme Inducers

These increase the activity of specific CYP enzymes over several days to weeks, leading to faster drug metabolism and reduced plasma concentrations of affected drugs (Table 1.4).

CYP450 Enzyme Inhibitors

These reduce the metabolic activity of CYP enzymes, leading to accumulation of drugs and increased risk of adverse effects (Table 1.5).

Special Note: Alcohol

Alcohol consumption has distinct effects on cytochrome P450 enzyme activity depending on the pattern of use. Acute alcohol intake inhibits CYP enzymes, particularly CYP2E1, which can reduce the metabolism of drugs reliant on this pathway (Lieber 1997). In contrast, chronic alcohol use induces CYP enzymes, most notably CYP2E1 and CYP3A4, leading to increased metabolic clearance of certain drugs and potential therapeutic failure (Zakhari 2013) (Table 1.6).

Table 1.4 CYP450 enzyme inducers

Common inducers	Mechanism/note
Carbamazepine	Strong CYP3A4 inducer, autoinduces its own metabolism
Phenytoin	Induces multiple CYPs, increases warfarin metabolism
Rifampicin	Potent CYP3A4 and P-gp inducer
Barbiturates	Especially phenobarbital
Smoking	Induces CYP1A2; affects clozapine, theophylline
Glucocorticoids	Induce several CYP enzymes
Griseofulvin	Antifungal with strong induction potential
St John's Wort	Herbal inducer of CYP3A4 and P-gp

Table 1.5 CYP450 enzyme inhibitors

Common inhibitors	Mechanism/Note
Metronidazole	Inhibits warfarin metabolism → ↑ INR
Ciprofloxacin	Inhibits CYP1A2
Fluconazole	Potent CYP2C9 and CYP3A4 inhibitor
Erythromycin/ clarithromycin	Inhibit CYP3A4 and prolong QT interval
Amiodarone	Inhibits multiple CYPs and P-gp
Cimetidine	H_2 receptor blocker with broad CYP inhibition
Ketoconazole	Strong CYP3A4 inhibitor
Etomidate	Inhibits adrenal steroidogenesis (not CYP3A4, but clinically relevant enzyme inhibition)
Grapefruit juice	Irreversible inhibitor of intestinal CYP3A4

Table 1.6 Examples of common interactions

Affected drug	Interaction	Clinical consequence
Warfarin	Inhibited by metronidazole/ erythromycin	↑ INR → bleeding risk
Midazolam	Inhibited by grapefruit juice	Prolonged sedation
OCP (ethinylestradiol)	Induced by rifampicin	Contraceptive failure
Fentanyl	Inhibited by fluconazole	Respiratory depression risk
Tacrolimus	Inhibited by macrolides	Nephrotoxicity, neurotoxicity

1.4 First and Zero Order Kinetics

Understanding how drugs are eliminated from the body is essential for safe and effective dosing. Drug elimination typically follows either first-order or zero-order kinetics, and the distinction has important implications for drug accumulation, toxicity, and dose adjustment.

First-Order Kinetics

Most drugs are eliminated from the body according to first-order kinetics, where the rate of drug elimination is directly proportional to the concentration of the drug in the plasma (Rowland and Tozer 2011a, b). In this scenario, a constant fraction of the drug is cleared per unit time. This means that the higher the plasma concentration, the faster the drug is metabolised and cleared. Under first-order conditions, the metabolic enzymes responsible for drug breakdown are not saturated; they are present in sufficient quantity to handle the available substrate. As a result, the half-life of the drug remains constant, regardless of the dose. This produces an exponential decline in drug concentration when plotted against time (Shargel et al. 2012a, b). Clinically, most anaesthetic and critical care agents follow first-order kinetics within their therapeutic range. Examples include paracetamol, propofol, fentanyl, and midazolam (Upton and Ludbrook 2005).

Zero-Order Kinetics

In contrast, zero-order kinetics describes a situation in which a constant amount of drug is eliminated per unit time, regardless of its plasma concentration. This occurs when the drug-metabolising enzymes become saturated, and their capacity to clear additional substrate has reached a maximum (Rowland and Tozer 2011a, b). Because the elimination rate is fixed, even small increases in dose can lead to disproportionate increases in plasma levels, increasing the risk of toxicity. Under zero-order kinetics, the half-life is variable and depends on the concentration of the drug. The decline in drug levels, when plotted against time, follows a linear pattern, rather than an exponential one (Shargel et al. 2012a, b). Classic examples of drugs that exhibit zero-order kinetics include ethanol (at all doses), phenytoin (within the therapeutic range), and aspirin (at high doses) (Levy 1994). Although warfarin is sometimes cited in older texts, it does not strictly follow zero-order kinetics; its metabolism is complex but largely first-order, with a long and variable half-life.

Clinical Relevance

The distinction between these two kinetic models is more than academic. Drugs with zero-order kinetics can accumulate rapidly and unpredictably, requiring careful monitoring and dose adjustment. This is particularly relevant in the perioperative and critical care settings, where altered physiology or hepatic function may further impair drug clearance (Rowland and Tozer 2011a, b) (Table 1.7).

Table 1.7 Comparison of first- and zero-order kinetics

Feature	First-order kinetics	Zero-order kinetics
Elimination pattern	Constant fraction per unit time	Constant amount per unit time
Rate of elimination	Proportional to plasma concentration	Independent of plasma concentration
Enzyme saturation	Enzymes not saturated	Enzymes saturated
Half-life (t½)	Constant	Varies with dose and concentration
Plasma concentration graph	Exponential decline	Linear decline
Clinical examples	Paracetamol, propofol, midazolam, fentanyl	Ethanol, phenytoin, aspirin (high dose)
Toxicity risk	Predictable accumulation	Higher risk of accumulation and toxicity

1.5 Isomers

Isomers are molecules that share the same molecular formula but differ in the arrangement of their atoms. This variation in structure can lead to significant differences in pharmacokinetic and pharmacodynamic properties, including potency, duration of action, metabolism, and side effect profile. Isomers are broadly classified into two main categories: structural isomers and stereoisomers.

Structural Isomers

Structural isomers, also called constitutional isomers, have the same molecular formula but differ in the connectivity of atoms, meaning the bonds between atoms are arranged differently (Eliel and Wilen 1994). These differences can produce molecules with similar, distinct, or even opposing physiological effects. A classic example is prednisolone and aldosterone, which are structural isomers with overlapping corticosteroid activity. Conversely, dihydrocodeine, an opioid analgesic, and dobutamine, a β_1-adrenergic agonist, are also structural isomers yet exhibit profoundly different pharmacological profiles (Testa and Krämer 2007).

Structural isomers can be further subdivided into the following categories:

1. Chain isomers—these differ in the arrangement of the carbon skeleton. While the functional group remains the same, changes to the carbon backbone may influence drug absorption and metabolism.
2. Positional isomers—these have the same carbon framework but the functional group is located at a different position on the molecule. This subtle shift can alter the drug's binding characteristics and activity.
3. Tautomeric isomers (tautomerism)—these are dynamic isomers that interconvert depending on environmental conditions such as pH. A clinically relevant example is midazolam, which exists in an open, ionised ring form at pH <4 (enhanc-

ing water solubility for ampoule formulation) and converts to a closed, unionised ring at pH >4, increasing lipid solubility and enabling it to cross the blood–brain barrier to exert sedative effects (Mandema et al. 1992).

Stereoisomers

Stereoisomers have the same molecular formula and atomic connectivity but differ in their three-dimensional spatial arrangement. These differences can profoundly affect how a drug interacts with its biological target, such as receptor binding or enzyme activity (Ariëns 1984).

Stereoisomers are classified into two main types:

1. **Optical isomers** (enantiomers and diastereoisomers)—optical isomers possess at least one chiral centre, typically a carbon atom bonded to four different groups. These isomers exist as non-superimposable mirror images, much like left and right hands, and rotate plane-polarised light in opposite directions but to the same extent. Enantiomers are mirror images of each other, while diastereoisomers are stereoisomers that are not mirror images. Despite chemical similarity, enantiomers may display markedly different pharmacological properties. For example, S-ketamine is more potent and produces fewer psychomimetic effects than R-ketamine (White et al. 1985), and levobupivacaine (the S-enantiomer of bupivacaine) has a lower cardiotoxicity profile than the racemic mixture (Foster and Markham 2000).
2. **Geometric isomers** (cis–trans isomers)—geometric isomers arise from restricted rotation around a double bond or within a rigid ring system. In cis-isomers, substituent groups are on the same side of the double bond, whereas in trans-isomers, they are on opposite sides. Although less commonly encountered in anaesthetic pharmacology, geometric isomerism is relevant in certain drug classes, including retinoids and some antihypertensive agents (Ariëns 1984).

1.6 Summary

Isomerism in pharmacology is a fundamental concept with important theoretical and practical implications. Although isomers share the same molecular formula, variations in the arrangement of atoms can lead to markedly different clinical effects. Isomers are broadly classified as either structural or stereoisomers. Structural isomers include chain, positional, and tautomeric forms, while stereoisomers comprise optical isomers—enantiomers and diastereoisomers—and geometric (cis–trans) isomers. Understanding these distinctions is critical when considering drug efficacy, safety, metabolism, and receptor selectivity, all of which are key considerations in anaesthesiology and critical care practice.

References

Ariëns, E.J. (1984) 'Stereochemistry, a basis for sophisticated nonsense in pharmacokinetics and clinical pharmacology', *European Journal of Clinical Pharmacology*, 26(6), pp. 663–668.

Bettler, B., Kaupmann, K., Mosbacher, J. and Gassmann, M. (2004) 'Molecular structure and physiological functions of GABA B receptors', *Physiological Reviews*, 84(3), pp. 835–867.

Brunton, L.L. (2018a) 'General principles of pharmacology', in Brunton, L.L., Hilal-Dandan, R. and Knollmann, B.C. (eds.) *Goodman & Gilman's The Pharmacological Basis of Therapeutics*. 13th edn. New York: McGraw-Hill, pp. 3–32.

Brunton, L.L. (2018b) 'Principles of toxicology and drug safety', in Brunton, L.L., Hilal-Dandan, R. and Knollmann, B.C. (eds.) *Goodman & Gilman's The Pharmacological Basis of Therapeutics*. 13th edn. New York: McGraw-Hill, pp. 65–78.

Calabrese, E.J. and Baldwin, L.A. (2003) 'The frequency of U-shaped dose responses in the toxicological literature', *Toxicological Sciences*, 62(2), pp. 330–338.

Changeux, J.P. (2012) 'Nicotinic acetylcholine receptors: from molecular biology to pathology', in Siegel, G.J., Albers, R.W., Brady, S.T. and Price, D.L. (eds.) *Basic Neurochemistry: Principles of Molecular, Cellular, and Medical Neurobiology*. 8th edn. Amsterdam: Elsevier, pp. 180–195.

Collingridge, G.L., Olsen, R.W., Peters, J. and Spedding, M. (2009) 'A nomenclature for ligand-gated ion channels', *Neuropharmacology*, 56(1), pp. 2–5.

Daly, J.W. (2000) 'Biochemical mechanisms of drug action: receptor regulation and signal transduction', in Pratt, W.B. and Taylor, P. (eds.) *Principles of Drug Action: The Basis of Pharmacology*. 4th edn. New York: Churchill Livingstone, pp. 85–110.

Eliel, E.L. and Wilen, S.H. (1994) *Stereochemistry of Organic Compounds*. New York: Wiley-Interscience, pp. 12–35.

Foster, R.H. and Markham, A. (2000) 'Levobupivacaine: a review of its pharmacology and use as a local anaesthetic', *Drugs*, 59(3), pp. 551–579.

Hilal-Dandan, R. and Brunton, L.L. (2018) 'Cellular signal transduction', in Brunton L.L., Hilal-Dandan, R. and Knollmann, B.C. (eds.) *Goodman & Gilman's The Pharmacological Basis of Therapeutics*. 13th edn. New York: McGraw-Hill, pp. 25–42.

Insel, P.A. (1996) 'Seminars in medicine of the Beth Israel Hospital, Boston. Adrenergic receptors—evolving concepts and clinical implications', *New England Journal of Medicine*, 334(9), pp. 580–585.

Katzung, B.G. and Vanderah, T.W. (2021) 'Drug receptors and pharmacodynamics', in Katzung, B.G. and Vanderah, T.W. (eds.) *Basic and Clinical Pharmacology*. 15th edn. New York: McGraw-Hill, pp. 31–44.

Kenakin, T. (2014) 'Pharmacological analysis of drug–receptor interactions', in Brunton, L.L., Chabner, B.A. and Knollmann, B.C. (eds.) *Goodman & Gilman's The Pharmacological Basis of Therapeutics*. 12th edn. New York: McGraw-Hill, pp. 35–60.

Lefkowitz, R.J. (1998) 'G protein-coupled receptors III. New roles for receptor kinases and β-arrestins in receptor signaling and desensitization', *Journal of Biological Chemistry*, 273(30), pp. 18677–18680.

Levy, G. (1994) 'Clinical pharmacokinetics of aspirin', *Pediatrics*, 93(3), pp. 516–519.

Levy, R.H., Thummel, K.E., Trager, W.F., Hansten, P.D. and Eichelbaum, M. (2000) *Metabolic Drug Interactions*. Philadelphia: Lippincott Williams & Wilkins.

Lieber, C.S. (1997) 'Cytochrome P-4502E1: its physiological and pathological role', *Physiological Reviews*, 77(2), pp. 517–544.

Lin, J.H. and Lu, A.Y.H. (1998) 'Role of pharmacokinetics and metabolism in drug discovery and development', *Pharmacological Reviews*, 50(4), pp. 475–514.

Lin, J.H. and Lu, A.Y.H. (2001) 'Interindividual variability in inhibition and induction of cytochrome P450 enzymes', *Annual Review of Pharmacology and Toxicology*, 41, pp. 535–567.

Mandema, J.W., Tuk, B., van Steveninck, A.L., Breimer, D.D. and Cohen, A.F. (1992) 'Pharmacokinetic–pharmacodynamic modeling of the central nervous system effects of midazolam and its main metabolite α-hydroxymidazolam in healthy volunteers', *Clinical Pharmacology & Therapeutics*, 51(6), pp. 715–728.

Neubig, R.R., Spedding, M., Kenakin, T. and Christopoulos, A. (2003) 'International Union of Pharmacology Committee on Receptor Nomenclature and Drug Classification. XXXVIII. Update on terms and symbols in quantitative pharmacology', *Pharmacological Reviews*, 55(4), pp. 597–606.

Olsen, R.W. and Sieghart, W. (2009) 'GABA A receptors: subtypes provide diversity of function and pharmacology', *Neuropharmacology*, 56(1), pp. 141–148.

Pelkonen, O., Turpeinen, M., Hakkola, J., Honkakoski, P., Hukkanen, J. and Raunio, H. (2008) 'Inhibition and induction of human cytochrome P450 enzymes: current status', *Archives of Toxicology*, 82(10), pp. 667–715.

Petrenko, A.B., Yamakura, T., Sakimura, K. and Baba, H. (2014) 'Defining the role of NMDA receptors in pain, analgesia, and anesthesia', *Anesthesia & Analgesia*, 118(4), pp. 915–933.

Rang, H.P. and Henderson, G. (2016) 'Cellular aspects of drug action', in Rang, H.P., Dale, M.M., Ritter, J.M., Flower, R.J. and Henderson, G. (eds.) *Rang and Dale's Pharmacology*. 8th edn. London: Churchill Livingstone, pp. 7–28.

Rowland, M. and Tozer, T.N. (2011a) *Clinical Pharmacokinetics and Pharmacodynamics: Concepts and Applications*. 4th edn. Philadelphia: Lippincott Williams & Wilkins, pp. 131–150.

Rowland, M. and Tozer, T.N. (2011b) *Clinical Pharmacokinetics and Pharmacodynamics: Concepts and Applications*. 4th edn. Philadelphia: Lippincott Williams & Wilkins, pp. 151–160.

Shargel, L., Wu-Pong, S. and Yu, A.B.C. (2012a) *Applied Biopharmaceutics and Pharmacokinetics*. 6th edn. New York: McGraw-Hill Medical, pp. 175–195.

Shargel, L., Wu-Pong, S. and Yu, A.B.C. (2012b) *Applied Biopharmaceutics and Pharmacokinetics*. 6th edn. New York: McGraw-Hill Medical, pp. 196–205.

Stockley, I.H. (2010) *Stockley's Drug Interactions*. 9th edn. London: Pharmaceutical Press.

Sutherland, E.W. (1972) 'Studies on the mechanism of hormone action', *Science*, 177(4047), pp. 401–408.

Testa, B. and Krämer, S.D. (2007) 'The biochemistry of drug metabolism – an introduction: Part 4. Reactions of conjugation and their enzymes', *Chemistry & Biodiversity*, 4(11), pp. 2571–2661.

Unwin, N. (2005) 'Refined structure of the nicotinic acetylcholine receptor at 4 Å resolution', *Journal of Molecular Biology*, 346(4), pp. 967–989.

Upton, R.N. and Ludbrook, G.L. (2005) 'Pharmacokinetic optimisation of intravenous anaesthesia', *Clinical Pharmacokinetics*, 44(1), pp. 5–20.

Vanderah, T.W. (2021) 'Drugs acting on cellular receptors and ion channels', in Katzung, B.G. and Vanderah, T.W. (eds.) *Basic and Clinical Pharmacology*. 15th edn. New York: McGraw-Hill, pp. 7–26.

White, P.F., Schüttler, J., Shafer, A., Stanski, D.R., Horai, Y. and Trevor, A.J. (1985) 'Comparative pharmacology of the ketamine isomers: studies in volunteers', *British Journal of Anaesthesia*, 57(2), pp. 197–203.

Wilkinson, G.R. (2005) 'Drug metabolism and variability among patients in drug response', *New England Journal of Medicine*, 352(21), pp. 2211–2221.

Zakhari, S. (2013) 'Alcohol metabolism and epigenetics changes', *Alcohol Research: Current Reviews*, 35(1), pp. 6–16.

Zanger, U.M. and Schwab, M. (2013) 'Cytochrome P450 enzymes in drug metabolism: regulation of gene expression, enzyme activities, and impact of genetic variation', *Pharmacology & Therapeutics*, 138(1), pp. 103–141.

Pharmacokinetics

2

2.1 Absorption and Bioavailability

Overview

Drug absorption refers to the process by which a drug moves from its site of administration into the bloodstream. Once in the systemic circulation, the drug becomes available to reach its target tissues. The rate and extent of absorption vary significantly depending on the drug's formulation, route of administration, physicochemical properties, and local physiological conditions (Amidon et al. 1995; Shargel et al. 2012a, b).

Factors Affecting the Rate of Drug Absorption

Several factors influence how rapidly and efficiently a drug is absorbed:

1. **Route of administration**—absorption rates vary depending on whether the drug is given intravenously, orally, sublingually, transdermally, or by another route.
2. **Molecular size**—smaller molecules cross biological membranes more readily than larger ones.
3. **pKa and ionisation**—only the unionised (lipid-soluble) form of a drug can cross lipid membranes efficiently. The extent of ionisation depends on the drug's pKa and the pH of the environment.
4. **Lipid solubility**—lipophilic drugs penetrate lipid-rich cell membranes more easily and tend to be absorbed more rapidly.
5. **Concentration gradient**—passive diffusion occurs down a concentration gradient, so higher drug concentrations at the site of administration can increase the rate of absorption (Table 2.1).

G. Browne, *PharmacologyPro*, https://doi.org/10.1007/978-3-032-10227-0_2

Table 2.1 Routes of drug administration

Route	Description	Key notes
Intravenous (IV)	Direct administration into systemic circulation	Bioavailability: 100% (F = 1.0)
Oral (Enteral)	Absorption through the gastrointestinal tract	Variable absorption; subject to first-pass metabolism
Intramuscular (IM)	Injection into muscle tissue	Absorption depends on blood flow, muscle mass, formulation
Transdermal	Through the skin	Steady absorption; requires lipophilic, potent drugs
Rectal	Via rectal mucosa	Partially avoids first-pass metabolism; useful if NPO
Sublingual/ Buccal	Under the tongue or against the cheek	Rapid absorption; bypasses first-pass metabolism
Inhalational	Via the respiratory tract	Rapid onset; used for local and systemic delivery
Intranasal	Through nasal mucosa	Rapid but variable absorption; bypasses first-pass metabolism
Epidural/ Intrathecal	Injected near or into the spinal cord	Regional effect; low systemic absorption
Vaginal	Via vaginal mucosa	Poor absorption overall; avoids first-pass metabolism

pKa and Ionisation

A drug's pKa is defined as the pH at which 50% of the drug exists in its ionised form and 50% remains unionised. This ionisation status is a critical determinant of drug absorption, as only the unionised form is sufficiently lipophilic to traverse cell membranes. The extent to which a drug is ionised depends on two key factors: the drug's intrinsic pKa and the pH of the surrounding environment. Acidic drugs, such as aspirin, are more readily absorbed in the acidic conditions of the stomach, while basic drugs like morphine are better absorbed in the more alkaline environment of the small intestine (Brodie et al. 1960). This concept is fundamental not only for understanding drug absorption but also for predicting the onset of action and distribution profiles of many anaesthetic agents (Williams et al. 2013).

Bioavailability

Bioavailability (F) refers to the proportion of an administered drug dose that reaches the systemic circulation in its unchanged form, and it is typically expressed as a percentage or decimal. For intravenous (IV) drugs, bioavailability is considered 100% (F = 1), as the drug is delivered directly into the bloodstream. In contrast, drugs administered via other routes—such as oral, rectal, or transdermal—often exhibit lower bioavailability due to factors like incomplete absorption and first-pass metabolism in the liver (Shargel et al. 2012a, b). Oral bioavailability is commonly assessed by comparing the area under the plasma concentration–time curve (AUC) following oral administration to the AUC after an IV dose of the same drug, using the formula: Bioavailability = (AUC_{oral} / AUC_{iv}) × 100% (Benet and Hoener 2002). Drugs with poor oral bioavailability may require alternative routes of administration or reformulation to achieve therapeutic effectiveness.

First-Pass Metabolism

First-pass metabolism refers to the initial hepatic metabolism of a drug before it reaches the systemic circulation. Drugs absorbed via the gastrointestinal tract first enter the portal venous system and pass through the liver, where they may be partially or extensively metabolised. This effect can significantly reduce the active concentration of the drug, lowering its systemic bioavailability (Wilkinson 1997). As a result, certain drugs (e.g. glyceryl trinitrate, morphine) are ineffective orally and require sublingual or parenteral administration. Understanding first-pass metabolism is critical when selecting the route of administration for drugs used perioperatively or in emergency settings (Lin and Lu 1997).

2.2 Drug Metabolism

Overview

Drug metabolism refers to the biochemical modification of pharmaceutical substances by living organisms, typically through specialised enzymatic systems. The primary aim of metabolism is to convert lipophilic drugs into more water-soluble metabolites, which can then be more easily excreted via the kidneys or in bile. The liver is the principal organ of drug metabolism, specifically within the smooth endoplasmic reticulum of hepatocytes. However, metabolism can also occur to a lesser extent in the gastrointestinal tract, lungs, kidneys, and skin (Guengerich 2008).

Phases of Hepatic Metabolism

Hepatic drug metabolism is classically divided into two sequential but distinct phases: Phase I (modification) and Phase II (conjugation).

Phase I Reactions—Modification

Phase I reactions are the initial metabolic processes that chemically modify a drug molecule, most commonly through oxidation, reduction, or hydrolysis. These reactions are primarily catalysed by the cytochrome P450 (CYP450) enzyme system (Guengerich 2001). The outcome of Phase I metabolism can vary depending on the drug: it may be inactivated, activated, or transformed into a reactive intermediate. For certain prodrugs, Phase I metabolism is essential to convert the inactive compound into its active therapeutic form—for example, enalapril undergoes Phase I metabolism to become enalaprilat, its active metabolite (Testa and Krämer 2008). If the resulting compound from Phase I is sufficiently polar, it may be eliminated directly via renal or biliary excretion without the need for further metabolic modification.

Phase II Reactions—Conjugation

Phase II metabolism involves the conjugation of a drug, or its Phase I metabolite, with a hydrophilic endogenous substrate to enhance water solubility and facilitate excretion. Common conjugation reactions in Phase II include glucuronidation, sulphation, acetylation, and methylation. While these reactions typically occur after Phase I metabolism, some drugs may bypass Phase I entirely and proceed directly to Phase II if they already possess suitable chemical groups for conjugation. The resulting conjugated compounds are usually pharmacologically inactive and are excreted predominantly via the urine or bile (King et al. 2000).

Factors Affecting Drug Metabolism

Drug metabolism varies considerably between individuals and patient populations due to physiological, genetic, and pathological factors.

Physiological factors—both neonates and elderly patients have reduced hepatic enzyme activity, which slows metabolism and increases the risk of drug accumulation. In neonates, immature glucuronidation pathways are particularly relevant for drugs such as chloramphenicol, which can lead to "grey baby syndrome" (Alcorn and McNamara 2002).

Genetic polymorphisms—variations in genes encoding drug-metabolising enzymes can result in individuals being classified as poor, intermediate, extensive, or ultra-rapid metabolisers. For example, codeine is a prodrug converted to morphine by CYP2D6; ultra-rapid metabolisers may produce toxic levels of morphine, while poor metabolisers may experience inadequate analgesia (Ingelman-Sundberg 2004). Similarly, suxamethonium metabolism depends on plasma cholinesterase (pseudocholinesterase), and individuals with atypical variants can develop prolonged neuromuscular blockade, a phenomenon known as suxamethonium apnoea (Kalow and Genest 1957).

Pathological states—liver disease impairs both Phase I and Phase II reactions, especially affecting drugs with high hepatic extraction ratios. Heart failure may reduce hepatic blood flow and delay drug clearance. Although renal dysfunction does not directly affect metabolism, it hampers the excretion of polar metabolites, leading to their accumulation (Verbeeck 2008).

Clinical Relevance in Anaesthesia and Critical Care

An understanding of hepatic drug metabolism is crucial in the perioperative setting, where rapid onset and offset of drugs, titratability, and minimisation of adverse effects are paramount. Conditions like hypoperfusion, multi-organ dysfunction, and polypharmacy can dramatically alter drug clearance, necessitating close monitoring and dose adjustments.

2.3 Half Life and Clearance

Volume of Distribution

The volume of distribution (VD) is a theoretical parameter that describes how extensively a drug distributes throughout the body's tissues relative to the plasma. It represents the volume in which the total amount of drug in the body would need to be uniformly distributed to achieve the observed plasma concentration, and is defined by the equation (Gibaldi and Perrier 1982):

$$VD = \text{Amount of drug in the body} / \text{Plasma drug concentration}$$

A low VD indicates that a drug remains largely within the intravascular space, suggesting minimal tissue penetration. Conversely, a high VD implies extensive distribution into peripheral tissues, fat stores, or intracellular compartments When the VD exceeds the total body water (~42 L in an adult), this reflects significant sequestration in tissues (Benet and Zia-Amirhosseini 1995).

Several factors influence the volume of distribution:

- **Lipid solubility**—lipophilic drugs, such as fentanyl and propofol, exhibit high VD due to widespread distribution into fat and tissue compartments.
- **Ionisation**—unionised drugs cross cell membranes more readily, contributing to a higher VD.
- **Plasma protein binding**—drugs that are highly bound to plasma proteins, such as warfarin, are confined largely to the vascular compartment, resulting in a lower VD.
- **Pathological states**—conditions such as renal failure increase total body water, expanding the apparent VD of hydrophilic drugs, while liver failure reduces plasma protein concentrations and oncotic pressure, increasing the VD of protein-bound drugs (Toutain and Bousquet-Mélou 2004).

The volume of distribution is expressed in litres (L) and is an important parameter for calculating drug dosing and clearance.

Half-Life ($t_{½}$)

The half-life (t½) of a drug is the time required for its plasma concentration to decrease by 50%. This is a fundamental concept in pharmacokinetics, as it informs dosing intervals, the time to reach steady state, and the duration of drug washout. In clinical practice, approximately 50% of the drug remains after one half-life, while about 96.9% is eliminated from plasma after five half-lives. This "five half-life rule" is commonly used to estimate the time required to reach steady state during continuous infusion or to predict the washout period after discontinuation (Rowland and Tozer 2011). Half-life is determined by both clearance (CL) and volume of distribution (VD), and can be calculated using the equation (Benet and Kroetz 2004):

$$t½ = 0.693 \times VD / CL$$

There is considerable variability in half-lives between drugs. For example, adenosine has an extremely short half-life of approximately 10 s, necessitating rapid intravenous bolus administration to achieve its effect, while amiodarone has a very long half-life of up to 110 days, which explains its prolonged therapeutic and adverse effects even after treatment is stopped (Zipes et al. 2006). The elimination kinetics of a drug—whether first-order or zero-order—also influence how its half-life behaves (Rowland and Tozer 2011).

Clearance (CL)

Clearance (CL) describes the efficiency with which a drug is removed from the plasma. It is defined as the volume of plasma completely cleared of the drug per unit time, and is typically expressed in millilitres per minute (mL/min) or litres per hour (L/h). Clearance can be calculated using the following equation (Wilkinson 2001):

$$\text{CL} = \text{Rate of elimination of drug} / \text{Plasma drug concentration}.$$

Clearance is a fundamental determinant of maintenance dosing, the duration of drug action, and the potential for drug accumulation during repeated dosing or continuous infusion. Drugs are cleared through several pathways, including hepatic metabolism, renal excretion, pulmonary elimination (as with volatile anaesthetics), and biliary clearance. It is important to distinguish between elimination and excretion: elimination refers to the removal of active drug from the plasma, encompassing both metabolism and distribution, while excretion refers specifically to the removal of the drug or its metabolites from the body, primarily via urine or bile (Davies and Morris 1993).

Interrelationship Between VD, Clearance, and Half-Life

These three pharmacokinetic parameters—clearance, volume of distribution, and half-life—are mathematically interdependent. An increase in volume of distribution generally prolongs the half-life, unless it is offset by a proportionate increase in clearance. Conversely, increased clearance shortens the half-life when the volume of distribution remains constant. Understanding these relationships is critical for clinical practice, as they underpin the calculation of an appropriate loading dose, which is determined by the volume of distribution, the maintenance infusion rate, which depends on clearance, and the time to reach steady state or achieve washout, which is governed by the half-life (Pang and Rowland 1977).

2.4 Compartment Models

Overview of Compartment Models

Compartment models are simplified mathematical frameworks used in pharmacokinetics to describe how a drug is absorbed, distributed, and eliminated in the body. Although the body is highly complex, compartment models allow us to estimate drug concentrations over time and guide appropriate dosing and administration frequency (Schnider and Shafer 2009). These models treat the body as a series of compartments in which a drug moves and is eventually eliminated. The most common are the one-compartment, two-compartment, and three-compartment models.

One-Compartment Model
The one-compartment model is the most basic and least physiologically accurate. It assumes that after a drug is administered, it instantly distributes uniformly throughout a single homogeneous compartment, which represents the entire body. From this compartment, the drug is eliminated by first-order kinetics, and plasma concentration declines in a mono-exponential fashion. When plotted on a semi-logarithmic graph, this yields a straight line. This model is useful for simpler drugs with limited distribution or for initial approximation of pharmacokinetics, but it underrepresents the distribution dynamics of most anaesthetic and critical care drugs (Schnider and Shafer 2009).

Two-Compartment Model
The two-compartment pharmacokinetic model adds complexity and more accurately reflects the behaviour of many clinically used drugs. In this model, the body is divided into a central compartment, representing the plasma and well-perfused organs such as the liver, kidneys, and lungs, and a peripheral compartment, representing less well-perfused tissues such as muscle and skin. Drugs are administered into and eliminated from the central compartment, but after administration they rapidly distribute between the central and peripheral compartments. This model accounts for two distinct phases in the plasma concentration–time profile: an initial distribution phase, during which the drug moves from the central to the peripheral compartment, and a subsequent elimination phase, in which the drug is cleared from the central compartment. The resulting plasma concentration–time curve follows a bi-exponential decay, characterised by a steep initial decline due to distribution, followed by a slower decline as elimination predominates (Hughes et al. 1992).

Three-Compartment Model
The three-compartment pharmacokinetic model is considered the most physiologically realistic, particularly for intravenous anaesthetic agents such as propofol, fentanyl, and thiopental. In this model, the body is divided into a central compartment, representing the blood and highly perfused organs such as the heart, lungs, liver, and kidneys; a rapidly equilibrating peripheral compartment, representing well-perfused tissues such as muscle; and a slowly equilibrating peripheral compartment, representing poorly perfused tissues such as fat and bone. Following administration, the drug distributes rapidly from the central compartment into well-perfused tissues, and more slowly into poorly perfused tissues. These peripheral compartments serve as reservoirs, from which the drug can later redistribute back into the plasma, particularly after infusion is stopped (Upton and Ludbrook 2005). The plasma concentration–time profile in this model is triphasic, comprising an initial rapid distribution phase (α-phase), a slower redistribution phase (β-phase), and a terminal elimination phase (γ-phase), which may be prolonged due to release of drug from fat stores. This model underpins the concept of context-sensitive half-time—a critical

consideration for drugs administered as prolonged infusions, where elimination depends not only on metabolism and clearance but also on the degree of saturation of the peripheral compartments (Hughes et al. 1992).

Clinical Relevance of Compartment Models

An understanding of compartment models is essential in clinical practice, as it informs the prediction of drug onset and duration of action, the determination of appropriate dosing intervals and infusion rates, and the anticipation of drug accumulation and delayed effects—particularly with lipophilic agents such as fentanyl and thiopental. These principles are also critical when tailoring dosing strategies for critically ill patients, whose altered perfusion, protein binding, and metabolism can significantly affect drug distribution and clearance. In anaesthetic practice, three-compartment models form the basis of target-controlled infusion (TCI) systems, which apply these pharmacokinetic principles to maintain stable plasma or effect-site drug concentrations during intravenous anaesthesia (Shafer and Gregg 1992; Anderson and Holford 2009).

Conflicts of Interest The authors have no conflicts of interest to declare that are relevant to the content of this chapter.

References

Alcorn, J. and McNamara, P.J. (2002) 'Pharmacokinetics in the newborn', *Advanced Drug Delivery Reviews*, 54(6), pp. 963–1017.

Amidon, G.L., Lennernäs, H., Shah, V.P. and Crison, J.R. (1995) 'A theoretical basis for a biopharmaceutic drug classification: the correlation of in vitro drug product dissolution and in vivo bioavailability', *Pharmaceutical Research*, 12(3), pp. 413–420.

Anderson, B.J. and Holford, N.H.G. (2009) 'Mechanism-based concepts of size and maturity in pharmacokinetics', *Annual Review of Pharmacology and Toxicology*, 49, pp. 303–327.

Benet, L.Z. and Hoener, B.A. (2002) 'Changes in plasma protein binding have little clinical relevance', *Clinical Pharmacology & Therapeutics*, 71(3), pp. 115–121.

Benet, L.Z. and Kroetz, D.L. (2004) 'Pharmacokinetics: The dynamics of drug absorption, distribution, metabolism, and elimination', in Goodman, L.S., Brunton, L.L., Lazo, J.S. and Parker, K.L. (eds.) *Goodman & Gilman's The Pharmacological Basis of Therapeutics*. 11th edn. New York: McGraw-Hill, pp. 29–48.

Benet, L.Z. and Zia-Amirhosseini, P. (1995) 'Basic principles of pharmacokinetics', *Toxicologic Pathology*, 23(2), pp. 115–123.

Brodie, B.B., Kurz, H. and Schanker, L.S. (1960) 'The importance of dissociation constant and lipid-solubility in influencing the passage of drugs into the stomach', *Journal of Pharmacology and Experimental Therapeutics*, 130(1), pp. 20–25.

Davies, B. and Morris, T. (1993) 'Physiological parameters in laboratory animals and humans', *Pharmaceutical Research*, 10(7), pp. 1093–1095.

Gibaldi, M. and Perrier, D. (1982) *Pharmacokinetics*. 2nd edn. New York: Marcel Dekker, pp. 45–68.

Guengerich, F.P. (2001) 'Common and uncommon cytochrome P450 reactions related to metabolism and chemical toxicity', *Chemical Research in Toxicology*, 14(6), pp. 611–650.

Guengerich, F.P. (2008) 'Cytochrome P450 and chemical toxicology', *Chemical Research in Toxicology*, 21(1), pp. 70–83.

Hughes, M.A., Glass, P.S. and Jacobs, J.R. (1992) 'Context-sensitive half-time in multicompartment pharmacokinetic models for intravenous anesthetic drugs', *Anesthesiology*, 76(3), pp. 334–341.

Ingelman-Sundberg, M. (2004) 'Pharmacogenetics of cytochrome P450 and its applications in drug therapy: the past, present and future', *Trends in Pharmacological Sciences*, 25(4), pp. 193–200.

Kalow, W. and Genest, K. (1957) 'A method for the detection of atypical forms of human serum cholinesterase: determination of dibucaine numbers', *Canadian Journal of Biochemistry and Physiology*, 35(4), pp. 339–346.

King, C.D., Rios, G.R., Green, M.D. and Tephly, T.R. (2000) 'UDP-glucuronosyltransferases', *Current Drug Metabolism*, 1(2), pp. 143–161.

Lin, J.H. and Lu, A.Y.H. (1997) 'Role of pharmacokinetics and metabolism in drug discovery and development', *Pharmacological Reviews*, 49(4), pp. 403–449.

Pang, K.S. and Rowland, M. (1977) 'Hepatic clearance of drugs. I. Theoretical considerations of a "well-stirred" model and a "parallel tube" model', *Journal of Pharmacokinetics and Biopharmaceutics*, 5(6), pp. 625–653.

Rowland, M. and Tozer, T.N. (2011) *Clinical Pharmacokinetics and Pharmacodynamics: Concepts and Applications*. 4th edn. Philadelphia: Lippincott Williams & Wilkins, pp. 161–178.

Schnider, T.W. and Shafer, S.L. (2009) 'Pharmacokinetics of intravenous anaesthetics', in Miller, R.D. (ed.) *Miller's Anesthesia*. 7th edn. Philadelphia: Churchill Livingstone, pp. 849–880.

Shafer, S.L. and Gregg, K.M. (1992) 'Algorithms to rapidly achieve and maintain stable drug concentrations at the site of drug effect with a computer-controlled infusion pump', *Journal of Pharmacokinetics and Biopharmaceutics*, 20(2), pp. 147–169.

Shargel, L., Wu-Pong, S. and Yu, A.B.C. (2012a) 'Drug absorption and bioavailability', in *Applied Biopharmaceutics and Pharmacokinetics*. 6th edn. New York: McGraw-Hill Medical, pp. 15–50.

Shargel, L., Wu-Pong, S. and Yu, A.B.C. (2012b) 'Bioavailability and bioequivalence', in *Applied Biopharmaceutics and Pharmacokinetics*. 6th edn. New York: McGraw-Hill Medical, pp. 51–78.

Testa, B. and Krämer, S.D. (2008) 'The biochemistry of drug metabolism – an introduction: Part 2. Redox reactions and their enzymes', *Chemistry & Biodiversity*, 5(11), pp. 2171–2336.

Toutain, P.L. and Bousquet-Mélou, A. (2004) 'Plasma clearance', *Journal of Veterinary Pharmacology and Therapeutics*, 27(6), pp. 415–425.

Upton, R.N. and Ludbrook, G.L. (2005) 'A physiologically based, recirculatory model of the kinetics and dynamics of propofol in man', *Anesthesiology*, 103(2), pp. 344–352.

Verbeeck, R.K. (2008) 'Pharmacokinetics and dosage adjustment in patients with hepatic dysfunction', *European Journal of Clinical Pharmacology*, 64(12), pp. 1147–1161.

Wilkinson, G.R. (1997) 'The hepatic drug clearance concept extended', *Clinical Pharmacology & Therapeutics*, 62(4), pp. 414–417.

Wilkinson, G.R. (2001) 'Pharmacokinetics: The dynamics of drug absorption, distribution, and elimination', in Hardman, J.G. and Limbird, L.E. (eds.) *Goodman & Gilman's The Pharmacological Basis of Therapeutics*. 10th edn. New York: McGraw-Hill, pp. 3–30.

Williams, D.A., Lemke, T.L. and Roche, V.F. (2013) 'Physicochemical properties of drugs: pKa and ionization', in Williams, D.A. and Lemke, T.L. (eds.) *Foye's Principles of Medicinal Chemistry*. 7th edn. Philadelphia: Lippincott Williams & Wilkins, pp. 51–76.

Zipes, D.P., Camm, A.J., Borggrefe, M., Buxton, A.E., Chaitman, B., Fromer, M., Gregoratos, G., Klein, G., Moss, A.J., Myerburg, R.J. and Priori, S.G. (2006) 'ACC/AHA/ESC 2006 guidelines for management of patients with ventricular arrhythmias and prevention of sudden cardiac death', *Journal of the American College of Cardiology*, 48(5), pp. e247–e346.

3 Cardiac Drugs

3.1 Anti-Arrhythmic Drugs

Introduction to Anti-arrhythmic Drugs

Anti-arrhythmic drugs are used to prevent or treat abnormal heart rhythms (arrhythmias), with the goal of restoring or maintaining normal sinus rhythm and controlling ventricular rate. These drugs are commonly used in the management of atrial fibrillation, atrial flutter, supraventricular tachycardias (SVTs), ventricular tachycardia (VT), and ventricular fibrillation (VF). In the anaesthetic and critical care setting, arrhythmias may occur perioperatively due to hypoxia, electrolyte imbalances, surgical manipulation, anaesthetic drugs, or underlying structural heart disease—making familiarity with anti-arrhythmic pharmacology essential (Zipes and Jalife 2014).

Classification of Anti-arrhythmic Drugs

The Vaughan–Williams classification, first proposed in the 1970s, remains the most widely used system for categorising anti-arrhythmic drugs (Vaughan Williams 1970). It groups agents according to their primary electrophysiological mechanism of action on the cardiac action potential. Despite its widespread use, the system has notable limitations. It is incomplete, as certain clinically important drugs such as adenosine, digoxin, and magnesium sulphate do not fit neatly into any class. There is considerable overlap of mechanisms, with drugs like amiodarone exhibiting effects across multiple classes (Singh and Hauswirth 1974). Furthermore, the classification is mechanistic rather than therapeutic, offering little insight into clinical indications, efficacy, or safety profiles. Landmark trials such as the Cardiac Arrhythmia Suppression Trial (CAST) highlighted the dangers of some Class I anti-arrhythmics, demonstrating increased mortality with encainide and flecainide despite suppression of ventricular ectopy (Echt et al. 1991). Nevertheless, the Vaughan–Williams classification continues to serve as a useful framework for understanding the pharmacodynamics of anti-arrhythmic agents.

G. Browne, *PharmacologyPro*, https://doi.org/10.1007/978-3-032-10227-0_3

The Vaughan–Williams Classification

The Vaughan–Williams classification divides anti-arrhythmic drugs into four main classes, with further subdivisions within Class I, based on their primary electrophysiological effects on the cardiac action potential.

- **Class I — sodium channel blockers**
- These agents inhibit fast sodium channels, predominantly affecting phase 0 depolarisation.
  - Class Ia — prolong the action potential duration and refractory period. Examples: quinidine, procainamide, disopyramide.
  - Class Ib — shorten the action potential duration and refractory period, particularly in depolarised or ischaemic tissue. Examples: lidocaine, phenytoin, mexiletine.
  - Class Ic — markedly slow conduction with minimal effect on refractory period. Examples: flecainide, propafenone.
- **Class II — beta-adrenergic blockers**
- These agents inhibit sympathetic stimulation, slowing nodal conduction and reducing heart rate. Examples: propranolol, metoprolol, esmolol, atenolol, bisoprolol.
- **Class III — potassium channel blockers**
- These drugs block potassium efflux during phase 3, prolonging repolarisation, action potential duration, and refractory period. Examples: amiodarone, sotalol, dofetilide, ibutilide.
- **Class IV — calcium channel blockers**
- These agents inhibit slow L-type calcium channels, primarily at the atrioventricular node, slowing conduction and prolonging refractory period. Examples: verapamil, diltiazem.

Other Important Agents (Unclassified by Vaughan–Williams)

Several clinically important agents do not fit neatly into the Vaughan–Williams classification. Adenosine produces transient atrioventricular nodal block through A_1 receptor activation and is first-line therapy for supraventricular tachycardia. Digoxin increases vagal tone and prolongs atrioventricular nodal refractoriness, making it useful for rate control in atrial fibrillation, particularly in heart failure. Magnesium sulphate is the treatment of choice for torsades de pointes and is also effective in digoxin-induced arrhythmias (January et al. 2014) (Table 3.1).

Table 3.1 Common arrhythmias and associated anti-arrhythmic agents used

Arrhythmia	Commonly used agents
Supraventricular tachycardia	Adenosine, verapamil, Beta-blockers, digoxin, Flecainide
Atrial fibrillation/ flutter	Beta-blockers, diltiazem, Digoxin (rate control); amiodarone, Flecainide, Propafenone (rhythm control); anticoagulation is also a key consideration
Ventricular tachycardia	Amiodarone, lidocaine, procainamide
Ventricular fibrillation	Amiodarone (after defibrillation), lidocaine
Torsades de pointes	Magnesium Sulphate
Digoxin toxicity	Phenytoin, magnesium, digoxin-specific antibody fragments (Digibind)

3.1.1 Amiodarone

Class

Amiodarone is primarily a Class III anti-arrhythmic agent according to the Vaughan–Williams classification. However, it also exhibits Class I (sodium channel blockade), Class II (beta-blockade), and Class IV (calcium channel blockade) effects, contributing to its broad anti-arrhythmic activity (Singh and Nademanee 1990).

Clinical Uses

Amiodarone is a highly versatile anti-arrhythmic agent, effective against a wide range of supraventricular and ventricular arrhythmias. It is indicated in the management of atrial fibrillation, atrial flutter, supraventricular tachycardia, ventricular tachycardia, and refractory ventricular fibrillation. It is also used in Wolff–Parkinson–White syndrome and for preventing recurrent arrhythmias in patients with structural heart disease or after myocardial infarction. Amiodarone is commonly employed in critical care and perioperative settings to control arrhythmias in unstable patients (Vassallo and Trohman 2007; Zimetbaum 2007).

Mechanism of Action

The principal anti-arrhythmic effect of amiodarone is blockade of cardiac potassium channels, which prolongs repolarisation, increases action potential duration, extends the effective refractory period, and suppresses re-entrant arrhythmias. In addition to its Class III effect, it inhibits sodium channels (slowing phase 0 depolarisation), exhibits non-competitive beta-blockade, and inhibits L-type calcium channels, contributing to its efficacy in both atrial and ventricular arrhythmias (Singh and Nademanee 1990).

Pharmacokinetics

Amiodarone displays complex pharmacokinetics. Oral bioavailability is variable and relatively low (~20–55%), and the drug is highly lipophilic with extensive tissue distribution and ~95% protein binding. It is metabolised hepatically via CYP3A4 and excreted primarily through bile, with minor elimination in tears and sweat. The terminal half-life is prolonged, averaging 58 days but ranging up to 142 days, leading to delayed steady-state concentrations and persistent pharmacological effects after discontinuation (Vassallo and Trohman 2007).

Adverse Effects

Amiodarone is associated with numerous and often serious adverse effects, which may involve nearly every organ system:

- **Cardiovascular:** QT prolongation with risk of torsades de pointes, bradycardia, hypotension (especially with intravenous use), and heart block.
- **Respiratory:** interstitial pneumonitis and pulmonary fibrosis, which can be fatal; baseline and serial chest imaging are recommended (Pollak 1999).
- **Hepatic:** liver enzyme elevation, hepatitis, cholestasis, and rarely cirrhosis; requires regular monitoring.
- **Thyroid:** both hypo- and hyperthyroidism due to iodine content and interference with hormone metabolism; monitor thyroid function periodically (Zimetbaum 2007).
- **Dermatological:** photosensitivity and slate-grey skin discolouration with chronic use.
- **Ophthalmological:** corneal microdeposits (usually asymptomatic) and, rarely, optic neuritis or neuropathy (Pollak 1999).
- **Neurological:** peripheral neuropathy, ataxia, tremor, and sleep disturbances.

Drug Interactions and Cautions

Amiodarone interacts with many drugs, increasing the risk of pro-arrhythmia when combined with other anti-arrhythmics and potentiating the effects of digoxin, warfarin, and statins through CYP inhibition and protein displacement. Caution is advised when used with other QT-prolonging agents such as fluoroquinolones, macrolides, and selective serotonin reuptake inhibitors. Peripheral vein irritation may occur with intravenous administration, so central access is preferred (Hilleman and Miller 1999).

Dosing

For acute intravenous management, a loading dose of 300 mg is given over 30–60 min, followed by a maintenance infusion of 900 mg over 24 h. Oral maintenance therapy is initiated at 200 mg three times daily for 1 week, then reduced to 200 mg twice daily for 1 week, and finally maintained at 200 mg once daily. Tapering is necessary to minimise tissue accumulation and toxicity (Vassallo and Trohman 2007).

Monitoring Parameters

Owing to its systemic toxicity, regular monitoring is essential. This includes thyroid and liver function tests, chest imaging (X-ray or computed tomography), ECG for QT prolongation, and ophthalmological assessment if visual symptoms develop (Hilleman and Miller 1999).

3.1.2 Digoxin

Class

Digoxin is a cardiac glycoside with both positive inotropic and atrioventricular (AV) nodal depressant effects (Hauptman and Kelly 1999).

Clinical Uses

Digoxin is used for its combined inotropic and chronotropic properties in two main clinical settings. It improves cardiac output in heart failure, particularly in patients with reduced ejection fraction and concurrent atrial fibrillation, by enhancing myocardial contractility. It is also employed for rate control in atrial fibrillation or flutter, particularly in sedentary patients or those with congestive heart failure where beta-blockers or calcium channel blockers are contraindicated. Although once used more broadly in heart failure, its role has diminished due to its narrow therapeutic index, lack of demonstrated mortality benefit, and risk of toxicity (Gheorghiade et al. 2006).

Mechanism of Action

Digoxin inhibits the Na^+/K^+-ATPase pump on the cardiac myocyte membrane, increasing intracellular sodium. This alters the activity of the Na^+/Ca^{2+} exchanger, leading to increased intracellular calcium and enhanced myocardial contractility (positive inotropy). In addition, inhibition of the Na^+/K^+-ATPase increases parasympathetic (vagal) tone, which reduces AV nodal conduction and slows the ventricular response in atrial fibrillation or flutter (Hauptman and Kelly 1999).

Pharmacokinetics

Digoxin is administered orally or intravenously, with high oral bioavailability (up to 80%) and low plasma protein binding (~25%). It undergoes minimal hepatic metabolism and is excreted largely unchanged in the urine, resulting in a half-life of approximately 30–45 h, which is prolonged in renal impairment. Dose adjustment in renal dysfunction is essential to prevent accumulation and toxicity (Gheorghiade et al. 2006).

Adverse Effects

Digoxin has a narrow therapeutic window, and toxicity is common, particularly in elderly patients or those with renal impairment, hypokalaemia, or interacting drugs such as amiodarone, verapamil, and macrolides.

- **Cardiovascular:** bradycardia, pro-arrhythmic effects including ventricular ectopy, paroxysmal atrial tachycardia with AV block, and junctional rhythms. Classic ECG changes include scooped ST segments ("Salvador Dalí sag" or "inverted tick sign"), shortened QT interval, prolonged PR interval, and flattened or inverted T-waves; these reflect digoxin effect but are not necessarily indicative of toxicity.
- **Gastrointestinal:** nausea, vomiting, anorexia.
- **Neurological and visual:** fatigue, confusion, blurred vision, xanthopsia (yellow or green halos), and red–green colour impairment.
- **Endocrine and other:** gynaecomastia and rash.

Toxicity and Antidote

Clinical toxicity is often observed at serum levels above 2.5 μg/L and can be fatal at levels exceeding 30 μg/L (Rathore et al. 2003). Management begins with stopping digoxin and supportive care, including atropine or pacing for bradycardia and correction of electrolyte disturbances, particularly potassium, magnesium, and calcium. In severe or life-threatening toxicity — manifesting as haemodynamic instability, ventricular arrhythmias, severe hyperkalaemia, or end-organ dysfunction — digoxin-specific antibody fragments (Digifab) may be administered. These bind circulating digoxin to form an inactive complex that is excreted in the urine. Digifab use is limited by its high cost and risk of serious adverse effects, including arrhythmias, electrolyte shifts, and anaphylaxis, and is generally reserved for severe toxicity (Gheorghiade et al. 2006).

Dosing

For acute loading, digoxin is administered as an intravenous infusion of 500 micrograms, followed by 250–500 micrograms after 6 h if needed. Maintenance oral dosing typically ranges from 62.5 to 500 micrograms once daily, with lower doses recommended in elderly patients, those with renal impairment, or low body weight. Serum levels should be checked after 5–7 days to ensure steady-state concentrations have been achieved (Rathore et al. 2003).

3.1.3 Verapamil

Class

Verapamil is a Class IV anti-arrhythmic agent and a non-dihydropyridine calcium channel blocker (Opie and Messerli 1990).

Primary Uses

Verapamil is used for the termination of paroxysmal supraventricular tachycardia (PSVT) and for rate control in atrial fibrillation and atrial flutter. It is also employed as an antihypertensive and for the management of angina pectoris, including variant

(Prinzmetal) angina. Less commonly, it may be used in migraine prophylaxis and hypertrophic cardiomyopathy (Echt and Cowan 1989).

Mechanism of Action

Verapamil inhibits L-type calcium channels, particularly in the sinoatrial and atrioventricular nodes, where conduction relies on calcium influx. This slows atrioventricular nodal conduction, prolongs the nodal refractory period, reduces heart rate, and decreases myocardial oxygen demand. As a vasodilator, it relaxes smooth muscle in the coronary and systemic arteries, contributing to its antihypertensive and antianginal effects. Verapamil primarily affects nodal tissue, with minimal impact on ventricular conduction in normal hearts (Opie and Messerli 1990).

Pharmacokinetics

Verapamil can be administered orally or intravenously. Oral bioavailability is approximately 20–35% due to high first-pass metabolism. Intravenous onset of action occurs within 1–5 min, and the elimination half-life ranges from 4 to 12 h, depending on age, liver function, and formulation. Verapamil is metabolised hepatically via CYP3A4 and exhibits nonlinear (zero-order) kinetics at high doses. Excretion is mainly renal in the form of metabolites, with only 3–4% excreted unchanged (Frishman et al. 2011).

Cautions and Contraindications

Verapamil should be avoided in heart failure with reduced ejection fraction, as it may worsen left ventricular function. In patients with Wolff–Parkinson–White syndrome and atrial fibrillation, it can accelerate conduction through the accessory pathway and precipitate ventricular fibrillation. Concomitant use with beta-blockers increases the risk of severe bradycardia, atrioventricular block, and asystole. It is contraindicated in significant hypotension, bradycardia, sick sinus syndrome, and second- or third-degree atrioventricular block in the absence of a pacemaker (Echt and Cowan 1989).

Adverse Effects

Common adverse effects include bradycardia, hypotension, worsening of left ventricular dysfunction, and constipation. Other reported effects are headache, dizziness, fatigue, peripheral oedema, and, rarely, elevated liver enzymes. Hypotension is more likely when given intravenously or combined with other vasodilators (Frishman et al. 2011).

Dosing

Oral verapamil is typically given at a total daily dose of 240–480 mg, divided into two or three doses or as an extended-release preparation. For acute PSVT termination, 5–10 mg may be administered by slow intravenous injection over 2 min (more slowly in elderly patients), with a second dose after 15–30 min if necessary. The usual maximum total intravenous dose is 20 mg (Opie and Messerli 1990).

3.1.4 Adenosine

Class

Adenosine is an endogenous purine nucleoside with potent anti-arrhythmic properties. It is not classified within the Vaughan–Williams system, but is often grouped separately due to its unique mechanism of action (DiMarco et al. 1983).

Clinical Uses

Adenosine is primarily indicated for the acute management of paroxysmal supraventricular tachycardia (PSVT), particularly in the termination of re-entrant supraventricular tachycardias involving the atrioventricular (AV) node, such as atrioventricular nodal re-entrant tachycardia (AVNRT) and atrioventricular re-entrant tachycardia (AVRT). It is also used diagnostically to differentiate supraventricular tachycardia from wide-complex tachycardias, such as ventricular tachycardia, by inducing transient AV nodal block and unmasking underlying atrial activity. In electrophysiology studies, adenosine can be used to assess sinus node function. It is ineffective in atrial fibrillation or flutter, though the transient slowing of AV nodal conduction can improve visualisation of atrial activity on the electrocardiogram (DiMarco et al. 1983).

Mechanism of Action

Adenosine binds to A1 receptors in the sinoatrial and atrioventricular nodes, which are G-protein–coupled receptors. This activates inhibitory Gi proteins, reducing cyclic AMP, opening potassium channels to hyperpolarise nodal tissue, and inhibiting L-type calcium channels. The result is a transient AV nodal block, interrupting re-entry circuits and restoring sinus rhythm in AV node–dependent tachycardias (Belardinelli et al. 1995).

Pharmacokinetics

Adenosine is administered exclusively as an intravenous bolus. It has an extremely short half-life of less than 10 s, with immediate onset of action. The drug is rapidly metabolised by adenosine deaminase in plasma and red blood cells, and eliminated through degradation to inosine followed by renal excretion. Because of its short half-life, it must be delivered as a rapid bolus into a large vein, followed immediately by a saline flush to ensure delivery to the heart before degradation (Belardinelli et al. 1995).

Adverse Effects

Adenosine is generally well tolerated due to its very short duration of action. However, patients often experience transient, intense symptoms that can be alarming, including flushing, chest discomfort, shortness of breath, palpitations, anxiety, and a characteristic sense of impending doom. Other notable adverse effects include bronchospasm, particularly in patients with asthma or chronic obstructive pulmonary disease, transient bradycardia or sinus pause, and rarely, hypotension or enhanced AV block, particularly in patients receiving beta-blockers or calcium channel blockers. Importantly, adenosine does not produce significant negative inotropic effects or sustained haemodynamic instability (DiMarco et al. 1983).

Dosing

Dosing follows Advanced Cardiac Life Support (ACLS) guidelines. The initial dose is 6 mg administered as a rapid intravenous bolus, followed immediately by a 20 mL saline flush. If ineffective within 1–2 min, a second dose of 12 mg may be administered, with a further 12 mg dose if necessary. Lower doses may be sufficient in patients with central venous access, those receiving dipyridamole, or heart transplant recipients due to enhanced sensitivity (Neumar et al. 2010).

3.1.5 Beta-Blockers

Class

Beta-blockers are β-adrenergic receptor antagonists that inhibit the effects of endogenous catecholamines. They can be categorised by their β1-selectivity (cardioselective versus non-selective), lipid solubility, presence of intrinsic sympathomimetic activity (ISA), and duration of action (Frishman 2003).

Clinical Uses

Beta-blockers are widely used across cardiovascular, neurological, and ophthalmic settings. Key indications include the management of hypertension, by reducing cardiac output and renin release, and secondary prevention after acute coronary syndrome, where they decrease myocardial oxygen demand and reduce arrhythmic risk. They are also used to control atrioventricular (AV) nodal–dependent tachyarrhythmias, such as atrial fibrillation and supraventricular tachycardia, and to treat heart failure with reduced ejection fraction (in selected agents). Other uses include migraine prophylaxis, anxiety management (particularly performance anxiety), essential tremor, and topical treatment of glaucoma with agents such as timolol (Bangalore et al. 2017).

Mechanism of Action

Beta-blockers antagonise β-adrenergic receptors in a tissue-specific manner. Blockade of β1-receptors in the heart and kidneys reduces heart rate, myocardial contractility, and renin secretion, while β2-receptor blockade in the lungs, vasculature, and metabolic tissues may lead to bronchospasm, peripheral vasoconstriction, and metabolic effects. Some agents are relatively β1-selective (e.g. metoprolol, bisoprolol, atenolol, esmolol), particularly at low doses, though this selectivity diminishes at higher doses. Certain beta-blockers exhibit intrinsic sympathomimetic activity, partially activating β-receptors while antagonising them, as seen with pindolol, which reduces bradycardia. Membrane-stabilising activity, observed with agents such as propranolol, has little clinical relevance (Cruickshank 2010).

Pharmacokinetics

Beta-blockers display variable pharmacokinetic properties. Highly lipid-soluble agents, such as propranolol and metoprolol, are well absorbed orally but undergo significant first-pass hepatic metabolism, cross the blood–brain barrier, and are cleared hepatically, contributing to central nervous system side effects. Poorly lipid-soluble agents, including atenolol and labetalol, have lower oral bioavailability, minimal central effects, and are excreted renally in largely unchanged form. Ultra–short-acting agents, such as esmolol, are metabolised rapidly by plasma esterases, have a half-life of approximately 9 min, and are particularly useful in perioperative and intensive care settings (Zipes et al. 2017).

Adverse Effects

Beta-blockers can produce a range of adverse effects. Cardiovascular effects include bradycardia, hypotension, AV block, reduced cardiac output (requiring caution in decompensated heart failure), and improved diastolic perfusion time, which may benefit coronary flow. Respiratory effects include bronchospasm, particularly in patients with asthma or chronic obstructive pulmonary disease; cardioselective agents mitigate but do not eliminate this risk. Neurological effects include fatigue, depression, nightmares, vivid dreams, and rarely hallucinations, particularly with lipid-soluble agents. Metabolic effects include masking of hypoglycaemic symptoms and alterations in lipid profiles, with increased triglycerides and reduced high-density lipoprotein cholesterol. Renal and endocrine effects include suppression of the renin–angiotensin–aldosterone system. Other effects include reduced intraocular pressure (topical use), dry mouth, and cold extremities due to peripheral vasoconstriction (Cruickshank 2010).

Clinical Considerations in Anaesthesia

Beta-blockers should generally be continued perioperatively to avoid rebound tachycardia and hypertension. Anaesthetists should monitor for bradycardia, particularly when combined with other AV nodal blocking agents such as calcium channel blockers or digoxin. Esmolol is particularly useful for acute heart rate control and blunting sympathetic surges during airway instrumentation. Initiation of beta-blockers should be avoided in patients with acutely decompensated heart failure (Zipes et al. 2017).

3.2 Antihypertensive Drugs

Overview

Antihypertensive drugs are a diverse group of agents used to lower arterial blood pressure and reduce cardiovascular risk, including stroke, myocardial infarction, and heart failure. They are used both in acute settings, such as perioperative hypertension or hypertensive crises, and in the chronic management of essential hypertension. Understanding the haemodynamic determinants of blood pressure is essential, as mean arterial pressure (MAP) is the product of cardiac output (CO) and systemic vascular resistance (SVR):

$$MAP = CO \times SVR$$

Cardiac output itself is determined by heart rate (HR) and stroke volume (SV):

$$CO = HR \times SV$$

Accordingly, antihypertensive agents lower blood pressure by reducing systemic vascular resistance (vasodilation), decreasing cardiac output (negative chronotropy or inotropy), or reducing preload and intravascular volume through diuresis (Brunton 2018; Whelton et al. 2018).

Classification of Antihypertensive Agents
Antihypertensives are generally classified by their primary mechanism of action. The main classes include vasodilators, diuretics (discussed in a separate chapter), beta-blockers, and centrally acting agents (Williams et al. 2018).

Vasodilators
Vasodilators are the principal class of antihypertensive drugs, acting by reducing SVR, often through vascular smooth muscle relaxation mediated by receptor or enzyme pathways. Subgroups include:

- **ACE inhibitors (ACEi):** inhibit angiotensin-converting enzyme, reducing angiotensin II and causing vasodilation (e.g. ramipril, enalapril) (Messerli et al. 2018).
- **Angiotensin II receptor blockers (ARBs):** directly antagonise angiotensin II receptors (e.g. losartan, candesartan).
- **Calcium channel blockers (CCBs):** inhibit L-type calcium channels in vascular smooth muscle (e.g. amlodipine) and cardiac tissue (e.g. verapamil).
- **Alpha-blockers:** antagonise α1-receptors, causing arterial and venous dilation (e.g. doxazosin).
- **Nitrates:** increase nitric oxide availability, leading to smooth muscle relaxation (e.g. glyceryl trinitrate [GTN]).
- **Sodium nitroprusside:** a potent, fast-acting arterial and venous dilator via nitric oxide release.
- **Hydralazine:** a direct arteriolar smooth muscle relaxant, particularly useful in pre-eclampsia.

Diuretics
Diuretics lower blood pressure by reducing intravascular volume and preload. Thiazides also exert a vasodilatory effect, reducing SVR. These agents are covered in detail in a separate chapter (Brunton 2018).

Beta-Blockers

Beta-blockers reduce blood pressure by lowering cardiac output through negative chronotropy and inotropy, and by inhibiting β1-receptors in the kidney, thereby suppressing renin release and attenuating the renin–angiotensin–aldosterone system (RAAS). They are particularly useful post-myocardial infarction and in patients with coexisting tachyarrhythmias, heart failure, or angina (Whelton et al. 2018).

Centrally Acting Agents

These agents lower blood pressure by reducing sympathetic outflow from the central nervous system, diminishing norepinephrine release at sympathetic nerve terminals. Examples include:

- **Clonidine:** an α2-agonist used for hypertensive urgency, withdrawal syndromes, and sedation.
- **Methyldopa:** an α2-agonist considered safe in pregnancy.
- **Ganglion blockers (e.g. trimetaphan):** rarely used, acting at nicotinic receptors in sympathetic ganglia.

Centrally acting agents are generally reserved for resistant hypertension or specific indications due to adverse effects such as sedation, dry mouth, and rebound hypertension (Brunton 2018).

Practical Considerations

In anaesthesia and critical care, antihypertensives should have rapid onset, be titratable, and possess short durations of action. Commonly used agents include GTN (for preload reduction), sodium nitroprusside (potent arterial and venous dilation), esmolol (ultra–short-acting β1-blocker for transient tachycardia or hypertension), and hydralazine (for severe hypertension or pre-eclampsia). For chronic outpatient management, long-acting oral agents are chosen based on patient-specific factors such as age, comorbidities, ethnicity, and tolerance. ACE inhibitors or ARBs are often preferred in younger patients and those with diabetes or heart failure, while calcium channel blockers are preferred in older or Afro-Caribbean patients (Flack et al. 2010; Williams et al. 2018). Beta-blockers are no longer first-line for primary hypertension but are appropriate when there is a compelling cardiac indication. Combination therapy is frequently required to achieve optimal blood pressure control (Whelton et al. 2018).

3.2.1 Calcium Channel Blockers

Class

Dihydropyridine calcium channel blockers (CCBs) are vasoselective agents that predominantly target vascular smooth muscle. They are chemically characterised as dihydropyridine derivatives, with commonly used examples including nifedipine, amlodipine, lercanidipine, and nimodipine (Abernethy and Schwartz 1999).

Overview

CCBs are broadly divided into two groups based on their predominant effects. Dihydropyridines act primarily on vascular smooth muscle, producing systemic vasodilation, while non-dihydropyridines (e.g. verapamil, diltiazem) exert more cardioselective effects, reducing nodal conduction and myocardial contractility. This section focuses on dihydropyridines, particularly nifedipine, which is widely used to lower systemic blood pressure and relax vascular smooth muscle (Frishman et al. 2011).

Clinical Uses

Dihydropyridine CCBs have a range of clinical applications, including:

- **Systemic hypertension** — for both acute and chronic control.
- **Angina pectoris** — by reducing afterload and improving coronary perfusion.
- **Raynaud's phenomenon** — via peripheral vasodilation.
- **Tocolysis** — to suppress premature uterine contractions.
- **High-altitude pulmonary oedema** — by lowering pulmonary artery pressure.
- **Cerebral vasospasm following subarachnoid haemorrhage** — nimodipine is specifically used to prevent delayed cerebral ischaemia (Pickard 2003).

Mechanism of Action

Dihydropyridine CCBs selectively inhibit L-type voltage-gated calcium channels on vascular smooth muscle, reducing intracellular calcium and decreasing muscle tone. This results in peripheral and coronary vasodilation, reduced systemic vascular resistance (SVR), and lower arterial pressure. Nifedipine may also exhibit weak mineralocorticoid receptor antagonism, though this is not clinically significant. Unlike non-dihydropyridines, dihydropyridines have minimal direct cardiac effects, although high doses or rapid-onset formulations (such as immediate-release nifedipine) may trigger reflex sympathetic activation and tachycardia (Opie 2004).

Pharmacokinetics

Dihydropyridines are administered orally and, in the case of Raynaud's phenomenon, occasionally topically. Intravenous use of nifedipine is avoided due to the risk of uncontrolled hypotension. Oral bioavailability is approximately 50% due to first-pass metabolism, and the drugs are metabolised hepatically via CYP3A4. The elimination half-life of immediate-release nifedipine is around 3.5 h but is longer for extended-release formulations. Excretion occurs via biliary and renal pathways (Frishman et al. 2011).

Adverse Effects

Dihydropyridines are generally well tolerated but can cause dose-dependent side effects:

- **Cardiovascular:** hypotension and reflex tachycardia, particularly with short-acting formulations, which may worsen angina by increasing oxygen demand.
- **Respiratory:** inhibition of hypoxic pulmonary vasoconstriction, which may exacerbate right-to-left shunting or pulmonary hypertension.
- **Neurological:** headache, dizziness, flushing, and increased cerebral blood flow (notably with nimodipine).
- **Other:** peripheral oedema (common), gingival hyperplasia (rare), and potentiation of neuromuscular blockade, which is relevant in anaesthesia (Opie 2004).

Precautions
Short-acting dihydropyridines, such as immediate-release nifedipine, are associated with marked reflex tachycardia and are generally avoided in acute coronary syndromes. These agents should also be used with caution in aortic stenosis, where reduced afterload may compromise coronary perfusion. Caution is advised with concomitant use of CYP3A4 inhibitors (e.g. macrolides, azoles), which can elevate plasma levels (Abernethy and Schwartz 1999).

Clinical Pearls
Long-acting formulations, such as amlodipine and extended-release nifedipine, are preferred for the chronic management of hypertension. Nimodipine is uniquely cerebroselective and improves neurological outcomes following subarachnoid haemorrhage by mitigating vasospasm (Pickard 2003). Unlike verapamil or diltiazem, dihydropyridine CCBs are not effective for rate control or the management of arrhythmias.

3.2.2 Angiotensin Receptor Blockers

Class
Angiotensin receptor blockers (ARBs) are angiotensin II type 1 (AT1) receptor antagonists that inhibit the actions of angiotensin II. Commonly used agents include losartan, olmesartan, valsartan, telmisartan, candesartan, and irbesartan (Burnier and Brunner 2000).

Clinical Uses
ARBs are widely prescribed for the management of systemic hypertension, heart failure, post-myocardial infarction (to reduce ventricular remodelling and improve survival), and left ventricular dysfunction. They are also used in diabetic nephropathy to reduce proteinuria and slow progression of chronic kidney disease (Parving et al. 2001). In anaesthetic practice, preoperative use of ARBs is common but carries important implications for intraoperative haemodynamic stability (Roshanov et al. 2017).

Mechanism of Action

ARBs selectively block AT1 receptors, preventing the vasoconstrictive, pro-fibrotic, and pro-hypertrophic effects of angiotensin II. This blockade produces systemic vasodilation by reducing systemic vascular resistance, decreases aldosterone secretion (resulting in reduced sodium and water retention), diminishes sympathetic outflow, and relieves efferent arteriolar constriction in the kidney, which can lower glomerular perfusion pressure. Unlike ACE inhibitors, ARBs do not inhibit bradykinin breakdown, which accounts for the lower incidence of dry cough and angioedema (Burnier and Brunner 2000).

Pharmacokinetics

ARBs are administered orally and have variable bioavailability (20–70%), depending on the specific agent. They are highly protein bound (>90%) and metabolised primarily in the liver, with losartan undergoing CYP2C9-mediated metabolism. Elimination occurs via mixed renal and biliary pathways. The half-life of most ARBs ranges from 5–15 h, but telmisartan has a prolonged half-life of up to 24 h, facilitating once-daily dosing (Burnier and Brunner 2000).

Adverse Effects

ARBs are generally well tolerated but can cause:

- **Hypotension**, particularly after the first dose or in hypovolaemic patients.
- **Hyperkalaemia** due to reduced aldosterone levels.
- **Renal impairment**, especially in patients with bilateral renal artery stenosis or advanced chronic kidney disease.
- **Gastrointestinal symptoms** such as nausea and diarrhoea.
- **Rare elevations in liver enzymes**.

In contrast to ACE inhibitors, dry cough is uncommon, and angioedema is significantly less frequent but remains possible (Burnier and Brunner 2000).

Perioperative Considerations

ARBs are associated with an increased risk of refractory hypotension under general anaesthesia, which may not respond adequately to catecholamines. They are therefore typically withheld 24 h before surgery. In cases of intraoperative hypotension, vasopressin or methylene blue may be required to restore vascular tone (Roshanov et al. 2017).

Other Notes

ARBs are generally more expensive than ACE inhibitors and should be initiated cautiously, particularly in volume-depleted patients, to avoid first-dose hypotension. They are particularly beneficial in diabetic nephropathy due to their nephroprotective effects (Parving et al. 2001).

Dosing

Dosing varies by agent and patient factors and should follow local guidelines. Typical starting doses include:

- **Losartan:** 50–100 mg once daily.
- **Telmisartan:** 20–80 mg once daily.
- **Valsartan:** 80–160 mg once or twice daily.

Clinical Pearl

ARBs provide cardiovascular and renal protection comparable to ACE inhibitors and are better tolerated in patients prone to cough or angioedema. Their long half-lives make them well suited for once-daily regimens, but careful titration and preoperative planning are necessary to minimise haemodynamic complications (McMurray et al. 2014).

3.2.3 Angiotensin-Converting Enzyme Inhibitors (ACEi)

Class

Angiotensin-converting enzyme inhibitors (ACE inhibitors) are renin–angiotensin–aldosterone system (RAAS) inhibitors that reduce the production of angiotensin II. Common agents include ramipril, captopril, lisinopril, perindopril, and enalapril (Dzau 2001).

Clinical Uses

ACE inhibitors are widely used in both acute and chronic settings for their cardiovascular and renal protective properties. Indications include systemic hypertension, post–acute coronary syndrome to limit ventricular remodelling and improve survival, chronic heart failure to reduce afterload and prolong life, and diabetic nephropathy to reduce proteinuria and slow the progression of kidney disease (Lewis et al. 1993; Yusuf et al. 2000). They are also used in patients with left ventricular dysfunction and occasionally for secondary stroke prevention in high-risk individuals (Yusuf et al. 2000).

Mechanism of Action

ACE inhibitors block the activity of angiotensin-converting enzyme, preventing the conversion of angiotensin I to angiotensin II, a potent vasoconstrictor. This results in vasodilation through reduced systemic vascular resistance, suppression of aldosterone release with consequent sodium and water loss, and diminished sympathetic outflow. In addition, ACE inhibition decreases bradykinin degradation, increasing its levels; this contributes to vasodilation but is also responsible for the dry cough and angioedema observed in some patients (Dzau 2001).

Pharmacokinetics

ACE inhibitors are administered orally and generally have good bioavailability (>70%), although absorption of some agents (e.g. captopril) may be reduced by food. They exhibit low plasma protein binding and are primarily metabolised in the liver to active forms, such as ramiprilat. Drugs in this class vary in half-life, with shorter-acting agents like captopril and enalapril requiring multiple daily doses, while longer-acting agents like ramipril and perindopril permit once-daily dosing. More than half of an administered dose is excreted unchanged in urine, and dose adjustments are required in renal impairment (Lewis et al. 1993).

Adverse Effects

ACE inhibitors are usually well tolerated, but notable adverse effects include:

- **Hypotension**, particularly with the first dose ("first-dose phenomenon").
- **Hyperkalaemia**, due to aldosterone suppression.
- **Dry, persistent cough**, affecting up to 20% of patients, attributed to bradykinin accumulation.
- **Renal impairment**, particularly in patients with bilateral renal artery stenosis.
- **Angioedema**, a rare but potentially life-threatening reaction, more common in Black and Afro-Caribbean patients (Yusuf et al. 2000).

Less frequent effects include taste disturbance, rash, leukopenia, thrombocytopenia, and gastrointestinal upset.

Perioperative Considerations

ACE inhibitors are generally withheld 24 h prior to elective surgery to reduce the risk of refractory intraoperative hypotension, which may not respond to standard catecholamines. In such cases, vasopressin or methylene blue may be required (Roshanov et al. 2017). First-dose hypotension can be minimised by initiating therapy at night, particularly in elderly or volume-depleted patients.

Other Notes

Although ACE inhibitors and ARBs have similar indications and efficacy, ACE inhibitors are more likely to cause cough and angioedema due to increased bradykinin levels. Combined use of an ACE inhibitor with an ARB is not recommended because of the elevated risk of renal dysfunction and hyperkalaemia (Lewis et al. 1993).

Dosing

Doses vary by agent and must be tailored to patient factors such as renal function, age, and concomitant therapy. Typical starting and maintenance doses include:

- **Ramipril:** 2.5–10 mg once daily.
- **Enalapril:** 5–20 mg twice daily.
- **Perindopril:** 4–8 mg once daily.

- **Captopril:** 12.5–50 mg two or three times daily.
- **Lisinopril:** 10–40 mg once daily.

Clinical Pearl
ACE inhibitors are cornerstone agents in cardiovascular and renal protection, particularly in patients with hypertension, diabetes, or heart failure. However, perioperative management requires careful planning to avoid haemodynamic instability (Roshanov et al. 2017).

3.2.4 Alpha-Blockers

Class Overview
Alpha-adrenergic antagonists, or alpha-blockers, inhibit the action of norepinephrine and epinephrine at alpha-adrenergic receptors, producing vasodilation and lowering systemic vascular resistance. They are classified by receptor selectivity:

- **Non-selective alpha-blockers** (e.g. phentolamine, phenoxybenzamine) block both α1 and α2 receptors.
- **Selective α1-blockers** (e.g. doxazosin, prazosin, tamsulosin) are predominantly used for hypertension and benign prostatic hyperplasia (BPH).
- **Selective α2-blockers** (e.g. yohimbine, mirtazapine) are rarely used in cardiovascular disease; mirtazapine is used as an antidepressant.

This section focuses on the clinically relevant selective α1-adrenergic blockers (Michel et al. 2006).

Clinical Uses
Alpha-blockers are used in both cardiovascular and urogenital indications. They are employed in hypertension, particularly resistant or refractory cases, although rarely as first-line therapy (Kaplan 2005). In BPH, they relax smooth muscle in the bladder neck and prostate to improve urinary outflow (Lepor 2007). Other indications include Raynaud's phenomenon, where vasodilation improves digital perfusion, and, occasionally, as adjuncts in congestive heart failure to reduce afterload. In the perioperative management of pheochromocytoma, phenoxybenzamine is used preoperatively to stabilise blood pressure (Bravo 2002). Phentolamine is occasionally used intracavernosally to treat erectile dysfunction.

Mechanism of Action
Alpha-blockers inhibit post-synaptic alpha-adrenergic receptors on vascular smooth muscle, reducing intracellular calcium and promoting relaxation. Blockade of α1 receptors interrupts Gq-protein signalling, decreasing inositol trisphosphate and diacylglycerol, and limiting calcium release from the sarcoplasmic reticulum. This leads to vascular smooth muscle relaxation and reduced systemic vascular

resistance. Non-selective agents also block α2 receptors, increasing norepinephrine release and sympathetic outflow, which can attenuate the antihypertensive effect (Michel et al. 2006).

Pharmacokinetics
Selective α1-blockers are administered orally, with good bioavailability high protein binding, and hepatic metabolism. Doxazosin has a long half-life (~22 h), allowing once-daily dosing, while prazosin has a shorter half-life (~3 h), requiring more frequent administration. Tamsulosin is selective for the α1A subtype in the prostate, producing minimal systemic hypotension (Lepor 2007).

Adverse Effects
Alpha-blockers are generally well tolerated, but side effects, especially with initial dosing, can be significant:

- **Cardiovascular:** first-dose hypotension (notably with prazosin), orthostatic hypotension, reflex tachycardia, and, rarely, QT prolongation.
- **Fluid and electrolyte:** sodium and water retention, potentially requiring a diuretic, and peripheral oedema.
- **Genitourinary:** retrograde ejaculation, particularly with tamsulosin, and urinary incontinence.
- **CNS:** dizziness, fatigue, and depression.
- **Other:** nasal congestion and dry mouth (Kaplan 2005; Lepor 2007).

Contraindications and Cautions
Alpha-blockers should be avoided or used with caution in patients with baseline hypotension, autonomic dysfunction, or volume depletion. Care is warranted when combined with other antihypertensives or vasodilators due to the risk of profound hypotension. Alpha-blockers may displace other protein-bound drugs such as warfarin and digoxin, necessitating monitoring of drug levels when applicable (Michel et al. 2006).

Clinical Pearls
Alpha-blockers should always be initiated at a low dose and titrated gradually to avoid the first-dose phenomenon, especially with prazosin. They are often combined with diuretics to counteract fluid retention. Tamsulosin is preferred in BPH because of its prostate selectivity and reduced hypotensive effects (Lepor 2007).

3.2.5 Clonidine

Class
Clonidine is a centrally acting α2-adrenergic receptor agonist with sympatholytic, sedative, and analgesic properties (Wallin and Sundlöf 1982).

Clinical Uses

Clonidine is a versatile drug used across anaesthesia, critical care, and chronic medicine. It is indicated for the management of hypertension, particularly resistant or rebound hypertension, and is widely employed perioperatively for sedation, anxiolysis, and haemodynamic stability. As an analgesic adjunct, it is added to epidural, spinal, or peripheral nerve blocks to enhance and prolong local anaesthetic effects and improve postoperative pain control (Eisenach et al. 1996). Clonidine is also used in the management of withdrawal syndromes, including opioids, benzodiazepines, and alcohol, and occasionally in paediatric attention deficit hyperactivity disorder. Its combination of sympatholytic, sedative, and analgesic effects makes it valuable in multimodal analgesia and enhanced recovery protocols (Kamibayashi and Maze 2000; Nishina and Mikawa 2002).

Mechanism of Action

Clonidine is a selective α2-adrenergic agonist that acts centrally and at the spinal level. In the brainstem, it stimulates α2-receptors to reduce sympathetic outflow, leading to decreased heart rate, reduced systemic vascular resistance, and lowered blood pressure (Wallin and Sundlöf 1982). In the dorsal horn of the spinal cord, it enhances the release of endogenous opioids and inhibits nociceptive transmission, contributing to its analgesic properties. Minimal action on α1-receptors reduces the risk of reflex tachycardia (Kamibayashi and Maze 2000).

Pharmacokinetics

Clonidine is administered via several routes, including oral, intravenous, transdermal, epidural, intrathecal, and as an adjunct in regional anaesthesia. It has high oral bioavailability (~100%), moderate protein binding (~30%), and is metabolised primarily in the liver to inactive metabolites, with renal excretion. The elimination half-life is approximately 14 h (range 6–20 h), and dose adjustment is recommended in renal impairment (Eisenach et al. 1996).

Adverse Effects

Clonidine is generally well tolerated but can cause:

- **Cardiovascular:** hypotension, particularly in hypovolaemic patients or with concurrent antihypertensives, bradycardia, and rebound hypertension if withdrawn abruptly.
- **Central nervous system:** sedation, fatigue, dizziness, and impaired concentration.
- **Other:** dry mouth, constipation, and sexual dysfunction.

When used neuraxially or in regional blocks, clonidine prolongs block duration and enhances analgesia but can cause hypotension and bradycardia (Eisenach et al. 1996).

Contraindications and Precautions

Abrupt withdrawal should be avoided to prevent rebound hypertension; tapering is recommended. Caution is advised in elderly patients, those with severe bradycardia, atrioventricular block, depression, or central nervous system disease (Kamibayashi and Maze 2000).

Dosage

Dosing depends on indication and route:

- **Systemic:** oral 0.2–0.6 mg/day in divided doses; transdermal patch 0.1–0.6 mg/24 h replaced weekly; intravenous 75–150 micrograms over 10–20 min.
- **Neuraxial:** epidural infusion 30 micrograms/hour; intrathecal (spinal) adjunct 15–30 micrograms added to local anaesthetic (Eisenach et al. 1996).

Clinical Pearls

Clonidine's ability to reduce opioid requirements, stabilise haemodynamics, and provide sedation makes it an important component of multimodal analgesia and enhanced recovery pathways. Its use as an adjunct in regional anaesthesia is increasing, given its ability to prolong block duration and improve postoperative analgesia with minimal systemic side effects when used in low doses (Kamibayashi and Maze 2000).

3.2.6 Sodium Nitroprusside

Class

Sodium nitroprusside (SNP) is a direct-acting vasodilator and nitric oxide (NO) donor with potent arterial and venous effects (Ignarro 1990).

Clinical Uses

SNP is used for the rapid control of blood pressure in critical and operative settings. Indications include intraoperative hypertension to manage acute hypertensive episodes and reduce bleeding, hypertensive emergencies in intensive care or emergency settings, and afterload reduction in severe heart failure or acute aortic regurgitation. Its use is restricted to monitored settings due to the risk of toxicity (Hall and Ward 1981).

Mechanism of Action

SNP releases nitric oxide, which activates guanylate cyclase in vascular smooth muscle, increasing intracellular cyclic GMP (cGMP). This lowers intracellular calcium, producing smooth muscle relaxation and potent vasodilation of both arterioles and venules. The combined reduction in systemic vascular resistance and venodilation decreases afterload and preload, lowering myocardial oxygen demand (Ignarro 1990).

Pharmacokinetics
SNP is administered exclusively by continuous intravenous infusion. Onset of action is rapid, within 30 s, and its effects dissipate within 1–2 min of stopping the infusion. It is metabolised in red blood cells to nitric oxide, cyanmethemoglobin, and cyanide ions. Cyanide is converted to thiocyanate in the liver by rhodanese and excreted renally. SNP itself has a short half-life of approximately 2 min, but thiocyanate may accumulate, especially in renal impairment, with a half-life of up to 3 days (Vesey and Cole 1985).

Adverse Effects
SNP is effective but associated with a range of adverse effects, particularly with high doses or prolonged infusions:

- **Cardiovascular:** profound hypotension, reflex bradycardia, catecholamine-mediated tachycardia, and reduced myocardial oxygen consumption.
- **Respiratory:** impaired hypoxic pulmonary vasoconstriction, worsening ventilation–perfusion mismatch.
- **Neurological:** headache, dizziness, confusion, restlessness, and increased intracranial pressure.
- **Gastrointestinal:** nausea and vomiting.
- **Metabolic:** tachyphylaxis and cyanide or thiocyanate toxicity (Vesey and Cole 1985).

Cyanide Toxicity
SNP metabolism releases cyanide, which inhibits mitochondrial cytochrome oxidase and impairs cellular respiration. Clinical features include metabolic acidosis, elevated venous oxygen content, tachycardia, dyspnoea, confusion, seizures, and, in severe cases, coma and cardiovascular collapse. Risk is increased with high doses (>2 mcg/kg/min for >24 h), or in renal or hepatic impairment. Monitoring should include blood gases, lactate, and oxygen saturation. Management involves stopping the infusion and administering antidotes: sodium thiosulfate, sodium nitrite, and hydroxocobalamin (Vesey and Cole 1985).

Other Considerations
SNP should only be administered via continuous intravenous infusion through a dedicated line with invasive arterial pressure monitoring. The solution must be protected from light to prevent degradation, and bolus dosing should be avoided to prevent abrupt hypotension (Hall and Ward 1981).

Dosage
Infusion is initiated at 0.5 mcg/kg/min and titrated every 5–10 min to a maximum of 6 mcg/kg/min, guided by haemodynamic response. The maximum recommended duration of infusion is typically less than 72 h (Dellinger et al. 2013).

Clinical Pearls
SNP's rapid onset and offset make it ideal for tightly controlled perioperative blood pressure management. However, the risk of cyanide toxicity limits its use in prolonged infusions, and alternative vasodilators with more favourable safety profiles, such as nicardipine or labetalol, are often preferred outside the operating room (Dellinger et al. 2013).

3.2.7 Glyceryl Trinitrate

Class
Glyceryl trinitrate (GTN) is an organic nitrate and direct vasodilator that donates nitric oxide (NO) to vascular smooth muscle (Abrams 1985).

Clinical Uses
GTN is a widely used vasodilator with potent venous and mild arteriolar effects, making it particularly useful in acute cardiovascular conditions. It is indicated for the relief and prophylaxis of angina pectoris, acute coronary syndromes including myocardial infarction, intraoperative or perioperative hypertension, and acute decompensated heart failure, particularly with pulmonary oedema. In anaesthesia and critical care, intravenous GTN is often employed to achieve controlled hypotension, reduce preload and afterload, lower myocardial oxygen demand, and improve pulmonary congestion (Levine et al. 2016).

Mechanism of Action
GTN is metabolised in vascular smooth muscle to release nitric oxide, which activates guanylate cyclase and increases intracellular cyclic GMP. This leads to reduced intracellular calcium, smooth muscle relaxation, and vasodilation. The predominant effect is venodilation, which decreases preload by reducing left ventricular end-diastolic volume and myocardial oxygen consumption, alleviating angina and pulmonary congestion. At higher doses, GTN also dilates arterioles, reducing afterload and further decreasing cardiac workload (Abrams 1985).

Pharmacokinetics
GTN can be administered sublingually, transdermally, or intravenously. Oral formulations are ineffective due to extensive first-pass metabolism. Onset of action is rapid — within 1–3 min for sublingual administration and immediate for intravenous infusion. Duration of action is 20–30 min for sublingual and ceases quickly after discontinuation of intravenous infusion. GTN is metabolised in the

liver and blood to dinitrate and mononitrate metabolites, which are excreted renally. The elimination half-life of the parent compound is approximately 3 min (Fung 2004).

Adverse Effects
GTN is generally well tolerated, but vasodilation may produce adverse effects:

- **Cardiovascular:** hypotension, orthostatic hypotension, reflex tachycardia, and syncope.
- **Neurological:** headache (common, due to cerebral vasodilation) and raised intracranial pressure, which can exacerbate intracranial pathology (Thadani and Lipicky 1983).

Precautions and Contraindications
GTN is contraindicated in patients taking phosphodiesterase-5 inhibitors (e.g. sildenafil, tadalafil) due to the risk of severe, prolonged hypotension and cardiovascular collapse (Levine et al. 2016). It should be used cautiously in hypovolaemia, severe anaemia, raised intracranial pressure, and glaucoma.

Tolerance
Tolerance may develop with chronic transdermal use, which can be mitigated by including nitrate-free intervals. No significant tolerance develops with short-term intravenous use (Fung 2004).

Dosage
- **Sublingual:** 400 micrograms per spray or tablet, repeated every 5 min as needed, up to three doses for angina.
- **Transdermal patch:** 5–10 mg over 24 h, applied to hairless skin and rotated to minimise irritation.
- **Intravenous infusion:** 1–10 mg/hour, titrated to effect with continuous monitoring of blood pressure and heart rate (Thadani and Lipicky 1983).

Clinical Pearls
GTN's rapid onset and short half-life make it ideal for precise haemodynamic control, particularly in the perioperative setting and in cardiogenic pulmonary oedema. It should be used cautiously in hypovolaemic patients to avoid worsening hypotension. Premedication with paracetamol may help reduce nitrate-induced headache (Fung 2004).

3.3 Vasopressors & Inotropes

Overview

Vasopressors and inotropes are cornerstone therapies in the management of shock and haemodynamic instability in critically ill and perioperative patients. Vasopressors induce vasoconstriction, increasing systemic vascular resistance (SVR) and raising mean arterial pressure (MAP), thereby improving perfusion to vital organs. Inotropes enhance cardiac contractility, increasing cardiac output (CO) and supporting circulatory flow. Although the term "inotrope" commonly refers to positive inotropic agents, negative inotropes, such as beta-blockers, also exist. Haemodynamic effects can be understood through the fundamental relationships:

$$\text{MAP} = \text{CO} \times \text{SVR}$$

$$\text{CO} = \text{Stroke Volume} \times \text{Heart Rate}.$$

Pharmacological modulation of any component of these equations influences perfusion pressure and organ blood flow (Cecconi et al. 2014; Levy et al. 2018).

Clinical Indications

Vasopressors and inotropes are primarily used in shock, defined as inadequate tissue perfusion resulting in cellular dysfunction. Shock is classified into four major types:

- **Hypovolaemic shock:** from volume loss (e.g. haemorrhage, severe dehydration).
- **Distributive shock:** from vasodilation and capillary leak (e.g. sepsis, anaphylaxis).
- **Cardiogenic shock:** from impaired cardiac pump function (e.g. myocardial infarction).
- **Obstructive shock:** from mechanical obstruction (e.g. massive pulmonary embolism, cardiac tamponade).

Pharmacological strategies differ by shock type. In distributive shock, vasopressors such as noradrenaline restore vascular tone and maintain MAP (Singer et al. 2016). In cardiogenic shock, inotropes such as dobutamine or milrinone improve contractility and output (De Backer et al. 2010). Hypovolaemic shock is managed primarily with fluid resuscitation, reserving vasopressors for persistent hypotension. In obstructive shock, treatment focuses on relieving the obstruction, with vasopressors providing supportive haemodynamics as needed (Cecconi et al. 2014).

Administration and Monitoring

Vasopressors and inotropes are administered intravenously, ideally via a central venous catheter to minimise the risk of extravasation and tissue necrosis. Continuous ECG and blood pressure monitoring are essential, with invasive arterial blood pressure monitoring recommended for precise titration. In selected intensive care settings, pulmonary artery catheters can be used to measure cardiac output, preload, and SVR. Frequent assessment of lactate, urine output, and end-organ function guides ongoing therapy (Dünser and Westphal 2008).

Clinical Pearls

Vasopressors and inotropes provide haemodynamic support but do not treat the underlying cause of shock, which must always be addressed. Therapy should begin with the lowest effective dose, titrated to achieve a target MAP, typically >65 mmHg in most patients. Excessive vasoconstriction can compromise perfusion of peripheral tissues, kidneys, and the gut. Combination therapy, such as noradrenaline with vasopressin, may lower individual drug doses and mitigate adverse effects. Tachyphylaxis may develop with some agents, notably metaraminol and phenylephrine, requiring close monitoring and dose adjustment (Levy et al. 2018) (Table 3.2).

3.3.1 Adrenaline

(Also known as epinephrine in North America)

Uses

Adrenaline is a potent sympathomimetic agent with combined vasopressor and inotropic properties, widely used in acute and critical care. It is the first-line treatment for anaphylaxis due to its α1-mediated vasoconstriction, β1-mediated positive inotropy, and β2-mediated bronchodilation (Simons et al. 2011). Adrenaline is a cornerstone of cardiac arrest management as part of Advanced Cardiac Life Support (ACLS) protocols (Nolan et al. 2015). It also provides inotropic support in low-output states, such as cardiogenic or septic shock, and is used as an adjunct to local

Table 3.2 Common vasopressors and inotropes

Drug	Class	Primary action
Noradrenaline (norepinephrine)	Vasopressor	α1 > β1 stimulation → ↑ SVR, modest ↑ HR
Phenylephrine	Vasopressor	Pure α1 agonist → ↑ SVR, reflex ↓ HR
Adrenaline (epinephrine)	Vasopressor/ inotrope	β1 > α1 > β2 → ↑ HR, CO, SVR
Vasopressin	Vasopressor	V1 agonist → potent vasoconstriction
Metaraminol	Vasopressor	Indirect sympathomimetic
Dobutamine	Inotrope	β1 > β2 agonist → ↑ contractility, CO
Milrinone	Inotrope	PDE-3 inhibitor → ↑ cAMP, vasodilation & inotropy

anaesthetics to reduce bleeding and prolong their effect through vasoconstriction (Dünser et al. 2009).

Mechanism of Action
Adrenaline is a non-selective adrenergic agonist, stimulating:

- **α1-receptors:** vasoconstriction, increasing systemic vascular resistance and blood pressure.
- **β1-receptors:** positive inotropy and chronotropy, increasing cardiac output.
- **β2-receptors:** bronchodilation and vasodilation in skeletal muscle.

This receptor profile makes adrenaline effective in reversing hypotension, relieving bronchospasm, and improving cardiac output in shock states (Barrett et al. 2019).

Pharmacokinetics
Adrenaline is rapidly metabolised by monoamine oxidase (MAO) and catechol-O-methyltransferase (COMT) in the liver, kidneys, and other tissues, forming metanephrine and normetanephrine, which are excreted renally. Its plasma half-life is short, approximately 2 min, necessitating repeated boluses or continuous infusion for sustained effect (Barrett et al. 2019).

Adverse Effects
Adrenaline's broad adrenergic activity produces systemic effects:

- **Cardiovascular:** tachycardia, increased contractility, elevated systemic vascular resistance, increased myocardial oxygen demand, with risks of arrhythmias and ischaemia.
- **Respiratory:** potent bronchodilation.
- **Neurological:** tremors, anxiety, headache, agitation.
- **Renal and splanchnic:** reduced perfusion to kidneys and gut.
- **Metabolic and endocrine:** hyperglycaemia and elevated lactate due to β2-mediated glycogenolysis and lipolysis, and increased renin–aldosterone activity (Dünser et al. 2009).

Other Considerations
Adrenaline infusions should be administered via a central venous line to avoid extravasation and tissue necrosis. It should be used cautiously in patients with ischaemic heart disease, hypertension, or pre-existing arrhythmias. β2-mediated glycolysis may exacerbate lactic acidosis in critically ill patients (Dünser et al. 2009).

Dosage

- **Cardiac arrest (ACLS):** 1 mg IV/IO every 3–5 min during resuscitation (Nolan et al. 2015).
- **Anaphylaxis:** 0.5 mg intramuscularly; alternatively, IV infusion in intensive care at 0.01–0.1 micrograms/kg/min, titrated to effect (Simons et al. 2011).
- **Perioperative hypotension:** boluses of 10–100 micrograms IV as needed.
- **Shock (infusion):** start at 0.01 micrograms/kg/min and titrate up to 0.1 micrograms/kg/min (Dünser et al. 2009).

3.3.2 Noradrenaline

(Also known as norepinephrine in North America)

Uses

Noradrenaline is the first-line vasopressor for the treatment of vasodilatory shock states. It is most commonly used in septic shock, neurogenic shock, and vasoplegia following cardiopulmonary bypass. By increasing systemic vascular resistance (SVR) and mean arterial pressure (MAP), noradrenaline improves perfusion to vital organs and stabilises haemodynamics in critically ill patients (Singer et al. 2016; De Backer et al. 2010).

Mechanism of Action

Noradrenaline is a potent α1-adrenergic agonist with modest β1 activity and negligible β2 effects.

- **α1-receptor activation:** produces arteriolar and venous vasoconstriction, increasing SVR and MAP.
- **β1-receptor activation:** at higher doses, confers mild positive inotropic and chronotropic effects, modestly increasing cardiac output.

Unlike adrenaline, noradrenaline does not cause significant bronchodilation or skeletal muscle vasodilation (Cecconi et al. 2014).

Pharmacokinetics

Noradrenaline is administered intravenously, ideally via a central venous catheter to prevent extravasation and tissue injury. It is rapidly metabolised by monoamine oxidase (MAO) in mitochondria and catechol-O-methyltransferase (COMT) in the cytoplasm. The primary metabolite, vanillylmandelic acid (VMA), is excreted in the urine. Its plasma half-life is short (approximately 2–3 min), necessitating continuous infusion (Cecconi et al. 2014).

Adverse Effects

- **Cardiovascular:** increased blood pressure, SVR, and pulmonary vascular resistance, with elevated myocardial oxygen demand from increased afterload.

- **Renal and splanchnic circulation:** reduced perfusion to the kidneys and gastrointestinal tract, particularly at high doses.
- **Local effects:** risk of extravasation injury and tissue necrosis if administered peripherally (Dünser and Hasibeder 2009).

Other Considerations
Noradrenaline is contraindicated in patients taking monoamine oxidase inhibitors (MAOIs) due to the risk of hypertensive crisis. It should be administered with continuous haemodynamic monitoring, ideally in a high-dependency or intensive care setting with an arterial line. In patients with concurrent low cardiac output, noradrenaline may be combined with an inotrope such as dobutamine to optimise haemodynamics (Cecconi et al. 2014).

Dosage
Noradrenaline is delivered by continuous intravenous infusion:

- **Starting dose:** 0.05–0.1 micrograms/kg/min.
- **Titration:** adjust in small increments to achieve haemodynamic targets.
- **Maximum:** doses up to 1 microgram/kg/min may be used in extreme cases, although high doses risk compromising end-organ perfusion (De Backer et al. 2010).

3.3.3 Ephedrine

Uses
Ephedrine is a sympathomimetic agent commonly used to treat hypotension and bradycardia in perioperative and emergency settings. It is particularly effective for managing anaesthesia-induced hypotension during spinal or general anaesthesia by increasing both blood pressure and heart rate (Baraka et al. 1997). Less commonly, ephedrine is used as a nasal decongestant, though this indication has declined due to systemic side effects and regulatory restrictions (Moran and Epstein 2006).

Mechanism of Action
Ephedrine exerts both direct and indirect sympathomimetic effects. It directly stimulates α- and β-adrenergic receptors, producing vasoconstriction (increasing systemic vascular resistance) and positive chronotropic and inotropic effects. Indirectly, it promotes the release of noradrenaline from presynaptic nerve terminals, enhancing adrenergic tone. Minimal inhibition of monoamine oxidase prolongs catecholamine activity but is not the primary mechanism. This mixed direct and indirect activity differentiates ephedrine from purely direct agents such as phenylephrine (Stoelting and Hillier 2006).

Pharmacokinetics
Ephedrine is typically administered intravenously in acute settings, although oral formulations are available. Oral bioavailability is high (~85%) but with a slower onset of action. Intravenous onset occurs within 1–2 min, with an elimination half-life of approximately 3 h. Ephedrine undergoes minimal hepatic metabolism and is excreted largely unchanged in the urine (Stoelting and Hillier 2006).

Adverse Effects
Ephedrine's adrenergic stimulation can produce several side effects:

- **Cardiovascular:** tachycardia, increased cardiac output, elevated blood pressure, and increased myocardial oxygen consumption, requiring caution in ischaemic heart disease.
- **Respiratory:** mild bronchodilation due to β_2 effects.
- **Renal:** transient reduction in glomerular filtration rate from vasoconstriction.
- **Other:** anxiety, tremor, and restlessness at higher doses (Butterworth et al. 2018).

Other Considerations
Tachyphylaxis to ephedrine can develop rapidly due to depletion of presynaptic noradrenaline stores, particularly after cumulative doses exceeding 30 mg (Butterworth et al. 2018). Its efficacy may be reduced in septic shock or catecholamine-depleted states, where reliance on endogenous noradrenaline limits its effectiveness. Unlike pure α-agonists such as phenylephrine, ephedrine increases both blood pressure and heart rate, making it safer for bradycardic hypotension (Baraka et al. 1997).

Dosage
Ephedrine is administered as intravenous boluses of 3–6 mg, repeated as necessary. Subsequent doses may need to be increased to overcome tachyphylaxis. Cumulative doses above 30–60 mg are generally avoided in most settings (Butterworth et al. 2018).

3.3.4 Phenylephrine

Uses
Phenylephrine is a selective α1-adrenergic agonist used primarily to manage hypotension during anaesthesia or in critical care by increasing systemic vascular resistance (SVR) and mean arterial pressure (MAP). It is also used topically as a nasal decongestant, to relieve haemorrhoidal symptoms, and to achieve mydriasis during ophthalmic procedures. Additional uses include reducing intraocular bleeding and treating priapism, where targeted vasoconstriction is beneficial (Morgan et al. 2013). In obstetric anaesthesia, phenylephrine is often preferred over ephedrine due to a lower risk of foetal acidosis (Ngan Kee et al. 2001; McDonnell and Paech 2007).

Mechanism of Action

Phenylephrine is a pure α1-adrenergic receptor agonist that produces vasoconstriction of both arterioles and veins, thereby increasing SVR and MAP. It has no β-adrenergic activity and thus does not directly increase heart rate or contractility. Reflex bradycardia may occur as a result of baroreceptor-mediated vagal activation in response to elevated blood pressure (Stoelting and Hillier 2006).

Pharmacokinetics

Phenylephrine can be administered intravenously, orally, intranasally, ophthalmically, or rectally. It is metabolised primarily in the liver by monoamine oxidase (MAO) and excreted renally. The onset of intravenous action is within minutes, with a duration of 15–20 min. Oral and topical effects may last up to 4 h (Stoelting and Hillier 2006).

Adverse Effects

Phenylephrine's vasoconstrictive effects can cause:

- **Cardiovascular:** reflex bradycardia, hypertension, and rarely arrhythmias.
- **Renal:** reduced renal perfusion due to vasoconstriction.
- **Neurological:** headache, anxiety, dizziness, and restlessness.
- **Local (topical):** nasal irritation and rebound congestion with prolonged use (Morgan et al. 2013).

Other Considerations

Reflex bradycardia is more pronounced in patients with intact vagal tone, such as young, healthy individuals. Phenylephrine should be used with caution in elderly, hypovolaemic, or cardiac patients. It is particularly useful in hypotensive patients with concomitant tachycardia, as it increases blood pressure without further elevating heart rate (McDonnell and Paech 2007).

Dosage

- **Intravenous bolus:** 50–100 micrograms, repeated as needed.
- **Intravenous infusion:** 20–50 micrograms per minute, titrated to effect.

Dosing should begin at the lower end and be increased cautiously, especially in elderly or hypertensive patients (Stoelting and Hillier 2006).

3.3.5 Dobutamine

Uses
Dobutamine is a synthetic catecholamine used primarily as an inotropic agent to augment cardiac output. It is indicated in low-output states such as cardiogenic shock, septic shock with myocardial dysfunction, and acute decompensated heart failure. Additionally, it is employed during cardiac stress testing in patients who cannot perform exercise-based tests due to physical limitations (Leier et al. 1977; Vincent and De Backer 2013).

Mechanism of Action
Dobutamine is a direct-acting β1-adrenergic agonist with minor β2 and α1 activity. Stimulation of β1 receptors increases myocardial contractility and heart rate, enhancing cardiac output. Mild β2-mediated vasodilation and α1-mediated vasoconstriction tend to offset each other, resulting in little net effect on systemic vascular resistance (SVR). Nonetheless, the vasodilatory component may lower blood pressure slightly, especially in hypovolaemic patients, and dobutamine is often combined with a vasopressor such as noradrenaline in hypotensive states (Tuttle and Mills 1975; Vincent and De Backer 2013).

Pharmacokinetics
Dobutamine is administered intravenously or intraosseously, with a rapid onset of action within 1–2 min. It has a short half-life of approximately 2 min and is metabolised in the liver and peripheral tissues by catechol-O-methyltransferase (COMT) to inactive metabolites, which are excreted in the urine (Tuttle and Mills 1975).

Adverse Effects
Dobutamine's sympathomimetic effects can lead to:

- **Cardiovascular:** tachycardia (dose-dependent), arrhythmias (particularly in patients with ischaemic heart disease), and hypotension from vasodilation in hypovolaemic states.
- **Other:** headache, nausea, and increased myocardial oxygen demand, which warrants caution in patients with coronary artery disease (Leier et al. 1977).

Increased urine output is often observed due to improved cardiac output and renal perfusion rather than a direct renal effect.

Other Considerations
Dobutamine should be used with caution in patients with atrial fibrillation or ventricular tachycardia due to its pro-arrhythmic potential. As it does not provide significant vasoconstriction, concomitant use of a vasopressor is often necessary in hypotensive patients. Continuous haemodynamic monitoring, ideally with arterial line and central venous access, is recommended during administration (Vincent and De Backer 2013). In chronic heart failure, prolonged catecholamine use such as

dobutamine has been associated with increased arrhythmias and mortality, limiting its long-term role (Packer et al. 1991).

Dosage

Dobutamine is given as a continuous infusion:

- **Initial dose:** 1 microgram/kg/min.
- **Titration:** increase gradually to achieve desired haemodynamic effect, with a typical range of 2–20 micrograms/kg/min.
- **Maximum dose:** up to 40 micrograms/kg/min in selected cases under intensive monitoring (Leier et al. 1977).

3.3.6 Vasopressin

(Also known as antidiuretic hormone, ADH)

Uses

Vasopressin is a non-catecholamine vasopressor used in the management of vasodilatory shock states, such as septic shock refractory to catecholamines, and post-cardiotomy vasoplegia (Russell et al. 2008). It has also been used in cardiac arrest (as per older ACLS guidelines), in the treatment of diabetes insipidus (using the desmopressin analogue), and, rarely, for controlling oesophageal variceal bleeding (Holmes et al. 2003).

Mechanism of Action

Vasopressin exerts its effects by acting on specific receptors:

- **V1a receptors (vascular smooth muscle):** mediates vasoconstriction, increasing systemic vascular resistance (SVR) and mean arterial pressure (MAP).
- **V2 receptors (renal collecting ducts):** promotes water reabsorption, expanding plasma volume and supporting blood pressure.
- **V1b receptors (anterior pituitary):** stimulates adrenocorticotropic hormone (ACTH) release, potentially supporting adrenal function in shock.

Unlike catecholamines, vasopressin does not depend on adrenergic receptors, making it particularly effective in refractory shock where adrenergic responsiveness is impaired (Landry et al. 1997; Holmes et al. 2003).

Pharmacokinetics

Vasopressin is administered intravenously (for shock) or intranasally/orally (for diabetes insipidus). Intravenous onset is within minutes, with a half-life of approximately 10–20 min. It is metabolised primarily by the liver and kidneys and excreted in the urine (Holmes et al. 2003).

Adverse Effects

Potential side effects include:

- **Cardiovascular:** excessive vasoconstriction, leading to peripheral or mesenteric ischaemia, bradycardia, and reduced cardiac output.
- **Renal:** hyponatraemia due to water retention via V2 activation.
- **Gastrointestinal:** nausea and abdominal cramps.
- **Cutaneous/peripheral:** skin blanching and digital ischaemia at higher doses (Dünser et al. 2003).

Other Considerations

Vasopressin is often used alongside noradrenaline in septic shock to allow catecholamine dose-sparing (Russell et al. 2008). Tachyphylaxis is uncommon compared to catecholamines. It should be avoided in patients with chronic hyponatraemia or ischaemic bowel disease. Monitoring should include serum sodium, urine output, and haemodynamics to prevent complications from water retention and ischaemia (Holmes et al. 2003).

Dosage

- **Vasodilatory shock:** continuous intravenous infusion at a fixed dose of 0.01–0.04 units/min, not titrated to effect like catecholamines (Russell et al. 2008).
- **Cardiac arrest (per older ACLS guidance):** a single intravenous bolus of 40 units as an alternative to 1 mg adrenaline (rarely used in contemporary practice).

Conflicts of Interest The authors have no conflicts of interest to declare that are relevant to the content of this chapter.

References

Abernethy, D.R. and Schwartz, J.B. (1999) 'Calcium-antagonist drugs', *New England Journal of Medicine*, 341(19), pp. 1447–1457.

Abrams, J. (1985) 'Mechanisms of action of the organic nitrates in the treatment of myocardial ischemia', *American Journal of Cardiology*, 56(8), pp. 12A–18A.

Bangalore, S., Steg, G., Deedwania, P., Crowley, K., Eagle, K.A., Goto, S., Ohman, E.M., Cannon, C.P., Smith, S.C., Zeymer, U., Hoffman, E., Messerli, F.H. and Bhatt, D.L. (2017) 'β-blocker use and clinical outcomes in stable outpatients with and without coronary artery disease', *JAMA*, 308(13), pp. 1340–1349.

Baraka, A., Taha, S. and Aouad, M. (1997) 'Comparison of phenylephrine and ephedrine in the treatment of hypotension during spinal anesthesia for cesarean section', *Anesthesia & Analgesia*, 84(2), pp. 376–380.

Barrett, K.E., Barman, S.M., Brooks, H.L. and Yuan, J.X.-J. (2019) *Ganong's Review of Medical Physiology*. 26th edn. New York: McGraw-Hill, pp. 261–265.

Belardinelli, L., Shryock, J.C. and Song, Y. (1995) 'Adenosine A1 receptors and the heart: actions, regulation, and therapeutic implications', *Circulation Research*, 76(3), pp. 415–423.

Bravo, E.L. (2002) 'Pheochromocytoma: an approach to antihypertensive management', *Annals of the New York Academy of Sciences*, 970(1), pp. 1–10.

Brunton, L.L. (2018) 'Antihypertensive agents', in Brunton, L.L., Hilal-Dandan, R. and Knollmann, B.C. (eds.) *Goodman & Gilman's The Pharmacological Basis of Therapeutics*. 13th edn. New York: McGraw-Hill, pp. 747–789.

Burnier, M. and Brunner, H.R. (2000) 'Angiotensin II receptor antagonists', *Lancet*, 355(9204), pp. 637–645.

Butterworth, J.F., Mackey, D.C. and Wasnick, J.D. (2018) *Morgan & Mikhail's Clinical Anesthesiology*. 6th edn. New York: McGraw-Hill, pp. 221–223.

Cecconi, M., De Backer, D., Antonelli, M., Beale, R., Bakker, J., Hofer, C., Jaeschke, R., Mebazaa, A., Pinsky, M.R., Teboul, J.L., Vincent, J.L. and Rhodes, A. (2014) 'Consensus on circulatory shock and hemodynamic monitoring. Task force of the European Society of Intensive Care Medicine', *Intensive Care Medicine*, 40(12), pp. 1795–1815.

Cruickshank, J.M. (2010) 'Beta-blockers continue to surprise us', *European Heart Journal*, 31(4), pp. 416–418.

De Backer, D., Biston, P., Devriendt, J., Madl, C., Chochrad, D., Aldecoa, C., Brasseur, A., Defrance, P., Gottignies, P. and Vincent, J.L. (2010) 'Comparison of dopamine and norepinephrine in the treatment of shock', *New England Journal of Medicine*, 362(9), pp. 779–789.

Dellinger, R.P., Levy, M.M., Rhodes, A., Annane, D., Gerlach, H., Opal, S.M., Sevransky, J.E., Sprung, C.L., Douglas, I.S., Jaeschke, R., Osborn, T.M., Nunnally, M.E., Townsend, S.R., Reinhart, K., Kleinpell, R.M., Angus, D.C., Deutschman, C.S., Machado, F.R., Rubenfeld, G.D., Webb, S.A., Beale, R.J., Vincent, J.L. and Moreno, R. (2013) 'Surviving Sepsis Campaign: international guidelines for management of severe sepsis and septic shock, 2012', *Intensive Care Medicine*, 39(2), pp. 165–228.

DiMarco, J.P., Sellers, T.D., Berne, R.M., West, G.A., Belardinelli, L., Berne, R.M. and Strauss, H.C. (1983) 'Adenosine: electrophysiologic effects and therapeutic use for terminating paroxysmal supraventricular tachycardia', *Circulation*, 68(6), pp. 1254–1263.

Dzau, V.J. (2001) 'Tissue renin–angiotensin system in myocardial hypertrophy and failure', *Archives of Internal Medicine*, 161(2), pp. 166–172.

Dünser, M.W. and Hasibeder, W.R. (2009) 'Sympathetic overstimulation during critical illness: adverse effects of adrenergic stress', *Journal of Intensive Care Medicine*, 24(5), pp. 293–316.

Dünser, M.W. and Westphal, M. (2008) 'Inotropes and vasopressors: an update', *Intensive Care Medicine*, 34(6), pp. 939–941.

Dünser, M.W., Mayr, A.J., Ulmer, H., Ritsch, N., Knotzer, H., Pajk, W., Luckner, G., Mutz, N.J. and Hasibeder, W.R. (2003) 'Arterial blood pressure during early sepsis and outcome', *Chest*, 123(4), pp. 1267–1273.

Dünser, M.W., Ruokonen, E., Pettilä, V., Ulmer, H., Torgersen, C., Schmittinger, C.A., Jakob, S.M., Takala, J. and Hasibeder, W.R. (2009) 'Association of arterial blood pressure and vasopressor load with septic shock mortality: a post hoc analysis of a multicenter trial', *Critical Care*, 13(6), R181.

Echt, D.S. and Cowan, J.C. (1989) 'Use of calcium antagonists in arrhythmias', *Circulation*, 80(5), pp. 1094–1106.

Echt, D.S., Liebson, P.R., Mitchell, L.B., Peters, R.W., Obias-Manno, D., Barker, A.H., Arensberg, D., Baker, A., Friedman, L., Greene, H.L., Huther, M.L. and Richardson, D.W. (1991) 'Mortality and morbidity in patients receiving encainide, flecainide, or placebo. The Cardiac Arrhythmia Suppression Trial', *New England Journal of Medicine*, 324(12), pp. 781–788.

Eisenach, J.C., De Kock, M. and Klimscha, W. (1996) 'Alpha2-adrenergic agonists for regional anesthesia: a clinical review of clonidine (1984–1995)', *Anesthesiology*, 85(3), pp. 655–677.

Flack, J.M., Sica, D.A., Bakris, G., Brown, A.L., Ferdinand, K.C., Grimm, R.H., Hall, W.D., Jones, W.E., Kountz, D.S., Lea, J.P., Nasser, S.A., Nesbitt, S.D., Saunders, E. and Scisney-Matlock,

M. (2010) 'Management of high blood pressure in Blacks: an update of the International Society on Hypertension in Blacks consensus statement', *Hypertension*, 56(5), pp. 780–800.

Frishman, W.H. (2003) 'Beta-adrenergic blockers: a 50-year historical perspective', *American Journal of Medicine*, 114(6), pp. 493–498.

Frishman, W.H., Cheng-Lai, A. and Nawarskas, J.J. (2011) 'Calcium channel blockers', in Mann, D.L., Zipes, D.P., Libby, P. and Bonow, R.O. (eds.) *Braunwald's Heart Disease: A Textbook of Cardiovascular Medicine*. 9th edn. Philadelphia: Saunders, pp. 841–863.

Fung, H.L. (2004) 'Pharmacokinetics and pharmacodynamics of organic nitrates: implications for clinical use', *Progress in Cardiovascular Diseases*, 47(2), pp. 93–109.

Gheorghiade, M., van Veldhuisen, D.J. and Colucci, W.S. (2006) 'Contemporary use of digoxin in the management of cardiovascular disorders', *Circulation*, 113(21), pp. 2556–2564.

Hall, V.A. and Ward, D.E. (1981) 'Sodium nitroprusside in anaesthesia and surgery', *British Journal of Anaesthesia*, 53(12), pp. 1249–1265.

Hauptman, P.J. and Kelly, R.A. (1999) 'Digitalis', in Zipes, D.P., Jalife, J. and Wellens, H.J.J. (eds.) *Cardiac Electrophysiology: From Cell to Bedside*. 3rd edn. Philadelphia: Saunders, pp. 1059–1070.

Hilleman, D.E. and Miller, M.A. (1999) 'Amiodarone: guidelines for use and monitoring', *American Family Physician*, 59(2), pp. 635–644.

Holmes, C.L., Landry, D.W. and Granton, J.T. (2003) 'Science review: Vasopressin and the cardiovascular system part 1—receptor physiology', *Critical Care*, 7(6), pp. 427–434.

Ignarro, L.J. (1990) 'Nitric oxide: a novel signal transduction mechanism for transcellular communication', *Annual Review of Pharmacology and Toxicology*, 30, pp. 535–560.

January, C.T., Wann, L.S., Alpert, J.S., Calkins, H., Cigarroa, J.E., Cleveland, J.C., Conti, J.B., Ellinor, P.T., Ezekowitz, M.D., Field, M.E., Murray, K.T., Sacco, R.L., Stevenson, W.G., Tchou, P.J., Tracy, C.M. and Yancy, C.W. (2014) '2014 AHA/ACC/HRS guideline for the management of patients with atrial fibrillation', *Circulation*, 130(23), pp. e199–e267.

Kaplan, N.M. (2005) 'Alpha-adrenergic blockers in the treatment of hypertension: is there a role?', *Journal of Hypertension*, 23(8), pp. 1441–1443.

Kamibayashi, T. and Maze, M. (2000) 'Clinical uses of alpha2-adrenergic agonists', *Anesthesiology*, 93(5), pp. 1345–1349.

Landry, D.W., Levin, H.R., Gallant, E.M., Ashton, R.C., Seo, S., D'Alessandro, D., Oz, M.C. and Oliver, J.A. (1997) 'Vasopressin deficiency contributes to the vasodilation of septic shock', *Circulation*, 95(5), pp. 1122–1125.

Leier, C.V., Webel, J. and Bush, C.A. (1977) 'The cardiovascular effects of dobutamine in patients with severe chronic heart failure', *American Journal of Medicine*, 63(2), pp. 306–312.

Lepor, H. (2007) 'Alpha blockers for the treatment of benign prostatic hyperplasia', *Reviews in Urology*, 9(4), pp. 181–190.

Levine, G.N., Bates, E.R., Bittl, J.A., Brindis, R.G., Fihn, S.D., Fleisher, L.A., Granger, C.B., Lange, R.A., Mack, M.J., Mauri, L., Mehran, R., Moussa, I.D., Mukherjee, D., Newby, L.K., O'Gara, P.T., Sabatine, M.S., Smith, P.K. and Smith, S.C. (2016) '2016 ACC/AHA guideline focused update on duration of dual antiplatelet therapy in patients with coronary artery disease', *Journal of the American College of Cardiology*, 68(10), pp. 1082–1115.

Levy, B., Buzon, J. and Kimmoun, A. (2018) 'Vasopressors in shock: a critical review', *European Journal of Anaesthesiology*, 35(4), pp. 245–253.

Lewis, E.J., Hunsicker, L.G., Bain, R.P. and Rohde, R.D. (1993) 'The effect of angiotensin-converting-enzyme inhibition on diabetic nephropathy', *New England Journal of Medicine*, 329(20), pp. 1456–1462.

McDonnell, N.J. and Paech, M.J. (2007) 'Phenylephrine and vasopressor choice during spinal anaesthesia for caesarean section', *Current Opinion in Anaesthesiology*, 20(4), pp. 321–325.

McMurray, J.J.V., Packer, M., Desai, A.S., Gong, J., Lefkowitz, M.P., Rizkala, A.R., Rouleau, J.L., Shi, V.C., Solomon, S.D., Swedberg, K. and Zile, M.R. (2014) 'Angiotensin–nepril-

sin inhibition versus enalapril in heart failure', *New England Journal of Medicine*, 371(11), pp. 993–1004.
Michel, M.C., Vrydag, W. and Korstanje, C. (2006) 'Alpha-adrenoceptor antagonists in clinical medicine: focus on the urinary tract', *British Journal of Clinical Pharmacology*, 61(6), pp. 661–675.
Messerli, F.H., Bangalore, S. and Bavishi, C. (2018) 'Angiotensin-converting enzyme inhibitors in hypertension: to use or not to use?', *Journal of the American College of Cardiology*, 71(13), pp. 1474–1482.
Moran, D.S. and Epstein, Y. (2006) 'Ephedrine, caffeine and performance', *Current Sports Medicine Reports*, 5(6), pp. 433–439.
Morgan, G.E., Mikhail, M.S. and Murray, M.J. (2013) *Clinical Anesthesiology*. 5th edn. New York: McGraw-Hill, pp. 227–229.
Neumar, R.W., Otto, C.W., Link, M.S., Kronick, S.L., Shuster, M., Callaway, C.W., Kudenchuk, P.J., Ornato, J.P., McNally, B., Silvers, S.M., Passman, R.S., White, R.D., Hess, E.P., Tang, W., Davis, D., Sinz, E. and Morrison, L.J. (2010) 'Part 8: Adult Advanced Cardiovascular Life Support: 2010 American Heart Association Guidelines for Cardiopulmonary Resuscitation and Emergency Cardiovascular Care', *Circulation*, 122(18 Suppl 3), pp. S729–S767.
Ngan Kee, W.D., Khaw, K.S., Tan, P.E., Ng, F.F. and Karmakar, M.K. (2001) 'Prophylactic phenylephrine infusion for preventing hypotension during spinal anesthesia for cesarean delivery', *Anesth Analg*, 93(3), pp. 708–713.
Nishina, K. and Mikawa, K. (2002) 'Clonidine in paediatric anaesthesia', *Current Opinion in Anaesthesiology*, 15(3), pp. 309–316.
Nolan, J.P., Soar, J., Cariou, A., Cronberg, T., Moulaert, V.R., Deakin, C.D., Bottiger, B.W., Friberg, H., Sunde, K. and Sandroni, C. (2015) 'European Resuscitation Council and European Society of Intensive Care Medicine guidelines for post-resuscitation care', *Intensive Care Medicine*, 41(12), pp. 2039–2056.
Opie, L.H. (2004) *Calcium Antagonists: Pharmacology and Clinical Research*. 2nd edn. Dordrecht: Springer.
Opie, L.H. and Messerli, F.H. (1990) 'Nondihydropyridine calcium antagonists: verapamil and diltiazem', *Journal of the American College of Cardiology*, 16(2), pp. 315–324.
Packer, M., Carver, J.R., Rodeheffer, R.J., Ivanhoe, R.J., DiBianco, R., Zeldis, S.M., Hendrix, G.H., Bommer, W.J., Elkayam, U., Kukin, M.L. and Mallis, G.I. (1991) 'Effect of oral milrinone on mortality in severe chronic heart failure', *New England Journal of Medicine*, 325(21), pp. 1468–1475.
Parving, H.H., Lehnert, H., Bröchner-Mortensen, J., Gomis, R., Andersen, S. and Arner, P. (2001) 'The effect of irbesartan on the development of diabetic nephropathy in patients with type 2 diabetes', *New England Journal of Medicine*, 345(12), pp. 870–878.
Pickard, J.D. (2003) 'Nimodipine in subarachnoid haemorrhage: a review after 20 years of clinical use', *Brain*, 126(7), pp. 1619–1631.
Pollak, P.T. (1999) 'Clinical organ toxicity of antiarrhythmic compounds: ocular and pulmonary manifestations', *American Journal of Cardiology*, 84(9A), pp. 37R–45R.
Rathore, S.S., Curtis, J.P., Wang, Y., Bristow, M.R. and Krumholz, H.M. (2003) 'Association of serum digoxin concentration and outcomes in patients with heart failure', *JAMA*, 289(7), pp. 871–878.
Roshanov, P.S., Rochwerg, B., Patel, A., Salehian, O., Duceppe, E., Belley-Cote, E., Guyatt, G.H., Sessler, D.I., Le Manach, Y., Borges, F.K., Tandon, V., Worster, A., Thabane, L., Paul, J., Devereaux, P.J. and POISE-2 Investigators (2017) 'Withholding versus continuing angiotensin-converting enzyme inhibitors or angiotensin II receptor blockers before noncardiac surgery', *Anesthesiology*, 126(1), pp. 16–27.
Russell, J.A., Walley, K.R., Singer, J., Gordon, A.C., Hébert, P.C., Cooper, D.J., Holmes, C.L., Mehta, S., Granton, J.T., Storms, M.M., Cook, D.J., Presneill, J.J. and Ayers, D. (2008) 'Vasopressin versus norepinephrine infusion in patients with septic shock', *New England Journal of Medicine*, 358(9), pp. 877–887.

Simons, F.E.R., Ardusso, L.R.F., Bilo, M.B., El-Gamal, Y.M., Ledford, D.K., Ring, J., Sanchez-Borges, M., Senna, G.E., Sheikh, A. and Thong, B.Y. (2011) 'World Allergy Organization guidelines for the assessment and management of anaphylaxis', *World Allergy Organization Journal*, 4(2), pp. 13–37.

Singh, B.N. and Hauswirth, O. (1974) 'Comparative mechanisms of action of antiarrhythmic drugs', *American Heart Journal*, 87(4), pp. 367–382.

Singh, B.N. and Nademanee, K. (1990) 'Amiodarone: historical development and pharmacologic profile', *American Heart Journal*, 120(4), pp. 1120–1138.

Singer, M., Deutschman, C.S., Seymour, C.W., Shankar-Hari, M., Annane, D., Bauer, M., Bellomo, R., Bernard, G.R., Chiche, J.D., Coopersmith, C.M., Hotchkiss, R.S., Levy, M.M., Marshall, J.C., Martin, G.S., Opal, S.M., Rubenfeld, G.D., van der Poll, T., Vincent, J.L. and Angus, D.C. (2016) 'The Third International Consensus Definitions for Sepsis and Septic Shock (Sepsis-3)', *JAMA*, 315(8), pp. 801–810.

Stoelting, R.K. and Hillier, S.C. (2006) *Pharmacology and Physiology in Anesthetic Practice*. 4th edn. Philadelphia: Lippincott Williams & Wilkins, pp. 309–314.

Thadani, U. and Lipicky, R.J. (1983) 'Clinical pharmacology of nitrates', *American Journal of Cardiology*, 52(7), pp. 14A–20A.

Tuttle, R.R. and Mills, J. (1975) 'Dobutamine: development of a new catecholamine to selectively increase cardiac contractility', *Circulation Research*, 36(1), pp. 185–196.

Vassallo, P. and Trohman, R.G. (2007) 'Prescribing amiodarone: an evidence-based review of clinical indications', *JAMA*, 298(11), pp. 1312–1322.

Vaughan Williams, E.M. (1970) 'Classification of antiarrhythmic drugs', *Pharmacology & Therapeutics. Part B: General and Systematic Pharmacology*, 1(1), pp. 115–138.

Vesey, C.J. and Cole, P.V. (1985) 'Sodium nitroprusside, cyanide, and thiocyanate', *Anaesthesia*, 40(8), pp. 775–785.

Vincent, J.L. and De Backer, D. (2013) 'Circulatory shock', *New England Journal of Medicine*, 369(18), pp. 1726–1734.

Wallin, B.G. and Sundlöf, G. (1982) 'Sympathetic outflow to muscles during clonidine therapy in essential hypertension', *Hypertension*, 4(5), pp. 715–721.

Whelton, P.K., Carey, R.M., Aronow, W.S., Casey, D.E., Collins, K.J., Dennison Himmelfarb, C., DePalma, S.M., Gidding, S., Jamerson, K.A., Jones, D.W., MacLaughlin, E.J., Muntner, P., Ovbiagele, B., Smith, S.C., Spencer, C.C., Stafford, R.S., Taler, S.J., Thomas, R.J., Williams, K.A., Williamson, J.D. and Wright, J.T. (2018) '2017 ACC/AHA/AAPA/ABC/ACPM/AGS/APhA/ASH/ASPC/NMA/PCNA guideline for the prevention, detection, evaluation, and management of high blood pressure in adults', *Journal of the American College of Cardiology*, 71(19), pp. e127–e248.

Williams, B., Mancia, G., Spiering, W., Rosei, E.A., Azizi, M., Burnier, M., Clement, D.L., Coca, A., de Simone, G., Dominiczak, A., Kahan, T., Mahfoud, F., Redon, J., Ruilope, L., Zanchetti, A., Kerins, M., Kjeldsen, S.E., Kreutz, R., Laurent, S., Lip, G.Y.H., McManus, R., Narkiewicz, K., Ruschitzka, F., Schmieder, R.E., Shlyakhto, E., Tsioufis, C., Aboyans, V. and Desormais, I. (2018) '2018 ESC/ESH Guidelines for the management of arterial hypertension', *European Heart Journal*, 39(33), pp. 3021–3104.

Yusuf, S., Sleight, P., Pogue, J., Bosch, J., Davies, R. and Dagenais, G. (2000) 'Effects of an angiotensin-converting–enzyme inhibitor, ramipril, on cardiovascular events in high-risk patients', *New England Journal of Medicine*, 342(3), pp. 145–153.

Zimetbaum, P. (2007) 'Amiodarone for atrial fibrillation', *New England Journal of Medicine*, 356(9), pp. 935–941.

Zipes, D.P. and Jalife, J. (2014) *Cardiac Electrophysiology: From Cell to Bedside*. 6th edn. Philadelphia: Elsevier Saunders, pp. 713–742.

Zipes, D.P., Jalife, J. and Stevenson, W.G. (2017) *Cardiac Electrophysiology: From Cell to Bedside*. 7th edn. Philadelphia: Elsevier, pp. 945–962.

4 Analgesics

4.1 NSAIDS

Overview

Non-steroidal anti-inflammatory drugs (NSAIDs) produce their analgesic, anti-inflammatory, and antipyretic effects primarily by inhibiting the cyclo-oxygenase (COX) enzyme, thereby reducing synthesis of inflammatory prostanoids—including prostaglandins, prostacyclin, and thromboxane (Vane and Botting 1998; Grosser et al. 2017). Arachidonic acid, derived from the cell membrane phospholipid bilayer via phospholipase A_2, can be metabolised through two pathways:

- **The COX pathway,** producing prostaglandins, prostacyclin, and thromboxane (collectively prostanoids).
- **The lipoxygenase pathway,** producing leukotrienes.

Inhibition of COX by NSAIDs shifts arachidonic acid metabolism towards increased leukotriene production, which may provoke bronchospasm in susceptible asthmatic patients (Vane and Botting 1998).

COX Isoforms

Cyclo-oxygenase exists in three isoforms with distinct physiological roles:

- **COX-1:** a constitutive enzyme expressed in most tissues, producing prostaglandins that maintain gastric mucosal integrity, renal blood flow, and platelet aggregation.
- **COX-2:** an inducible enzyme upregulated at sites of inflammation, responsible for pain, fever, and swelling.
- **COX-3:** a variant of COX-1 found in the central nervous system and thought to mediate some effects of paracetamol, though its clinical significance remains under investigation (Warner and Mitchell 2004).

G. Browne, *PharmacologyPro*, https://doi.org/10.1007/978-3-032-10227-0_4

COX-2 selective inhibitors (e.g. celecoxib, etoricoxib) were developed to maintain anti-inflammatory and analgesic benefits while minimising gastrointestinal toxicity. However, their use has been associated with increased cardiovascular risk, including myocardial infarction and stroke (Bombardier et al. 2000).

Prostanoids and Their Functions

The clinical effects of prostanoids are diverse. Prostaglandin E_2 (PGE_2) plays a protective role in the gastrointestinal tract by safeguarding the gastric mucosa and inhibiting gastric acid secretion. Prostacyclin (PGI_2) acts as a potent vasodilator and also inhibits platelet aggregation, contributing to vascular homeostasis. In contrast, prostaglandin $F_2\alpha$ ($PGF_2\alpha$) promotes bronchoconstriction and uterine contraction, making it relevant in respiratory and obstetric physiology. Thromboxane A_2 exerts opposing effects by promoting platelet aggregation and vasoconstriction, thereby playing a key role in haemostasis (Moncada and Vane 1979; Vane and Botting 1995).

Clinical Uses

Non-steroidal anti-inflammatory drugs (NSAIDs) are widely used in clinical practice for a variety of indications. They provide effective analgesia in cases of mild-to-moderate pain, particularly when of musculoskeletal origin. Their anti-inflammatory properties make them useful in the management of conditions such as arthritis and tendonitis. NSAIDs are also employed as antipyretic agents to reduce fever in febrile illnesses. In the perioperative setting, they form an important component of multimodal analgesia strategies, helping to minimise opioid requirements and improve overall pain control (Grosser et al. 2017).

Adverse Effects

NSAID use is associated with several important adverse effects:

- **Gastrointestinal:** COX-1 inhibition reduces mucosal protection, increasing the risk of gastritis, ulceration, and gastrointestinal bleeding (Bombardier et al. 2000).
- **Renal:** inhibition of prostaglandin-mediated renal vasodilation may precipitate acute kidney injury, particularly in hypovolaemic or elderly patients (Grosser et al. 2017).
- **Cardiovascular:** COX-2 inhibitors disrupt the prostacyclin–thromboxane balance, predisposing to thrombotic events such as myocardial infarction and stroke (Bombardier et al. 2000).
- **Respiratory:** increased leukotriene production can exacerbate bronchospasm, especially in asthmatic patients (Vane and Botting 1995).
- **Haematological:** inhibition of thromboxane A_2 impairs platelet aggregation, prolonging bleeding time (Patrono et al. 2017).

Contraindications

NSAIDs should be avoided or used with caution in patients with:

- Known NSAID or aspirin hypersensitivity.
- Asthma with prior NSAID-induced bronchospasm.
- Renal impairment or congestive heart failure.
- Active or previous gastrointestinal ulceration or bleeding.
- Coagulation disorders or concomitant anticoagulant therapy.
- Age <15 years (aspirin contraindicated due to risk of Reye's syndrome).
- Concomitant warfarin therapy, as NSAIDs displace warfarin from protein-binding sites, increasing bleeding risk (Grosser et al. 2017; Patrono et al. 2017) (Table 4.1).

Table 4.1 Comparison of common NSAIDs

Drug	COX selectivity	Half-life	Route(s)	Metabolism	Key clinical notes
Ibuprofen	Non-selective COX	2–4 h	Oral, IV	Hepatic (CYP2C9)	Widely used. Fewer GI side effects than some others. Lower cardiovascular risk. Common first-line NSAID
Naproxen	Non-selective COX	12–17 h	Oral	Hepatic (CYP1A2, CYP2C9)	Longer-acting. Lower cardiovascular risk compared to other non-selective NSAIDs
Aspirin	Irreversible COX-1 > 2	3–20 h (dose-dependent)	Oral	Hepatic & plasma esterases	Antiplatelet at low doses. Contraindicated in children (Reye's syndrome). Can cause significant GI toxicity
Diclofenac	COX-2 > COX-1	1–2 h	Oral, topical, rectal	Hepatic (CYP2C9)	Higher cardiovascular risk. Available in topical forms for localised pain (e.g., osteoarthritis)

(continued)

Table 4.1 (continued)

Drug	COX selectivity	Half-life	Route(s)	Metabolism	Key clinical notes
Indomethacin	Non-selective COX	4–5 h	Oral, rectal, IV	Hepatic	Potent anti-inflammatory. Higher risk of CNS side effects (headache, dizziness). Often used for gout
Ketorolac	Non-selective COX	4–6 h	IV, IM, oral, intranasal	Hepatic	Strong analgesic, comparable to opioids. High risk of GI bleeding—use limited to ≤5 days
Meloxicam	COX-2 > COX-1 (semi-selective)	15–20 h	Oral, IV	Hepatic (CYP2C9, CYP3A4)	Long-acting. Better tolerated GI-wise than non-selective NSAIDs
Celecoxib	Selective COX-2	11 h	Oral	Hepatic (CYP2C9)	Lower GI toxicity. Increased cardiovascular risk. Used cautiously in patients with atherosclerotic disease
Etoricoxib	Highly selective COX-2	22 h	Oral	Hepatic (CYP3A4)	Long-acting. Good for chronic conditions (e.g. arthritis). Avoid in patients with established cardiovascular or cerebrovascular disease

4.1.1 Aspirin

Overview

Aspirin (acetylsalicylic acid) is a non-selective, irreversible cyclo-oxygenase (COX) inhibitor with analgesic, anti-inflammatory, antipyretic, and prominent antiplatelet effects. Its role in cardiovascular prophylaxis has made it one of the most widely prescribed medications worldwide (Vane and Botting 2003; Patrono et al. 2005).

Uses

Aspirin has a broad range of clinical uses. It is primarily indicated for antiplatelet therapy, particularly in the secondary prevention of myocardial infarction (MI), ischaemic stroke, and transient ischaemic attack (TIA) (Antithrombotic Trialists' Collaboration 2002; Patrono et al. 2005). It also provides effective analgesia for mild-to-moderate pain, especially of musculoskeletal or inflammatory origin. As an anti-inflammatory agent, aspirin is used in conditions such as rheumatoid arthritis. It serves as an antipyretic to reduce fever in adults. Additionally, aspirin is used in settings such as percutaneous coronary intervention (PCI), in patients with low-risk non-valvular atrial fibrillation, and as part of dual antiplatelet therapy (Patrono et al. 2005).

Mechanism of Action

Aspirin irreversibly inhibits COX-1 and COX-2 enzymes by acetylating a serine residue in their active sites.

- **COX-1 inhibition** in platelets suppresses thromboxane A_2 (TXA_2) production, reducing platelet aggregation and vasoconstriction. As platelets lack nuclei, they cannot synthesise new COX enzymes, making aspirin's antiplatelet effect last for the lifespan of the platelet (7–10 days) (Vane and Botting 2003).
- **COX-2 inhibition** mediates analgesic, anti-inflammatory, and antipyretic effects, but also contributes to systemic side effects (Grosser et al. 2006).

Pharmacokinetics

Aspirin is rapidly absorbed in the stomach and upper small intestine, with an oral bioavailability of approximately 80% and high protein binding (~80%) It is metabolised primarily in the liver and extra-hepatic tissues via esterases to salicylic acid, which is further conjugated to inactive metabolites. At low doses, elimination follows first-order kinetics, but at higher doses or overdose it shifts to zero-order kinetics, increasing the risk of accumulation. The elimination half-life is approximately 3 h at low doses and up to 20 h at higher doses (Patrono et al. 2005).

Adverse Effects

- **Gastrointestinal:** gastric ulceration and bleeding due to reduced mucosal protection (Vane and Botting 2003).
- **Renal:** decreased renal perfusion and fluid retention, particularly in the elderly and those with pre-existing renal disease.
- **Respiratory:** bronchospasm in susceptible asthmatic patients due to increased leukotriene production.
- **Cardiovascular:** generally haemodynamically neutral but may exacerbate heart failure by promoting fluid retention (Grosser et al. 2006).
- **Other:** tinnitus (early sign of salicylate toxicity), rare hepatic dysfunction (Proudfoot and Krenzelok 2010).

Special Considerations

- **Protein binding:** aspirin competes with other highly protein-bound drugs such as warfarin, potentially increasing their free concentration and risk of bleeding (Patrono et al. 2005).
- **Reye's syndrome:** a rare but serious complication of acute encephalopathy and liver failure in children under 15 years, particularly during viral illness. Aspirin is contraindicated in paediatric patients unless under specialist guidance (Vane and Botting 2003).
- **Overdose:** presents with mixed respiratory alkalosis and metabolic acidosis, tinnitus, and potentially coma. Management includes urine alkalinisation, supportive care, and dialysis in severe cases (Proudfoot and Krenzelok 2010).

Dosage

- **Antiplatelet prophylaxis:** 75 mg once daily for long-term secondary prevention.
- **Acute thrombotic event:** 300 mg stat loading dose.
- **Analgesic/anti-inflammatory:** 300–600 mg every 4–6 h.
- **Maximum daily dose:** 4 g in divided doses (Antithrombotic Trialists' Collaboration 2002; Patrono et al. 2005)

4.1.2 Paracetamol

Uses

Paracetamol is a widely used analgesic and antipyretic. It is a first-line agent for mild-to-moderate pain and is often employed as part of multimodal analgesia regimens to reduce opioid requirements, particularly in the perioperative and critical care settings (Prescott 2000).

Mechanism of Action

The exact mechanism of paracetamol remains incompletely understood. It is thought to act primarily through central inhibition of cyclo-oxygenase-3 (COX-3) and modulation of central serotonergic pathways. Unlike non-steroidal anti-inflammatory drugs (NSAIDs), paracetamol has minimal anti-inflammatory activity and does not significantly inhibit peripheral COX enzymes (Graham and Scott 2005).

Pharmacokinetics

Paracetamol is well absorbed orally, with bioavailability around 80%. It exhibits low protein binding (~10%) and is primarily metabolised in the liver by glucuronidation and sulphation pathways. A small fraction is metabolised by cytochrome P450 (mainly CYP2E1) to produce a toxic intermediate metabolite. The drug and its conjugated metabolites are excreted renally. The elimination half-life is approximately 2 h in healthy adults but may be prolonged in overdose or hepatic impairment (Forrest et al. 1982).

Adverse Effects

Paracetamol is generally well tolerated but can cause:

- Hepatotoxicity in overdose due to accumulation of the toxic metabolite N-acetyl-p-benzoquinone imine (NAPQI).
- Hypotension and bradycardia with rapid intravenous administration.
- Rare haematological complications, including immune thrombocytopaenic purpura.
- Hypersensitivity reactions such as rash and, rarely, Stevens–Johnson syndrome (Prescott 2000).

Toxicity and Antidote

In therapeutic doses, the small amount of NAPQI formed is detoxified by hepatic glutathione. In overdose, glutathione stores become depleted, allowing NAPQI to accumulate and cause potentially fatal hepatocellular necrosis. The antidote, N-acetylcysteine (NAC), replenishes glutathione and limits liver damage. Management of overdose is guided by serum paracetamol concentration and time since ingestion, typically using the Rumack–Matthew nomogram (Rumack 2002; Heard 2008).

Dosage

- Adults ≥50 kg: 1 g every 6 h (maximum 4 g per day).
- Adults <50 kg or frail/elderly: 15 mg/kg every 6 h (maximum 60 mg/kg/day or 3 g per day).
- Paediatrics: 15 mg/kg every 4–6 h, not exceeding 60 mg/kg/day without specialist guidance (Prescott 2000).

4.2 Opioids

Overview

Opioids are a class of drugs that produce their effects by binding to opioid receptors in the central and peripheral nervous systems as well as the gastrointestinal tract. The term encompasses natural opiates (e.g. morphine, codeine), derived from the opium poppy, as well as semi-synthetic derivatives (e.g. oxycodone, hydromorphone) and fully synthetic compounds (e.g. fentanyl, methadone, tramadol). Opioids remain among the most effective treatments for moderate-to-severe pain but are limited by the development of tolerance, physical dependence, and a broad range of side effects (Benyamin et al. 2008).

Opioid Receptors

Opioid receptors are G-protein–coupled receptors traditionally classified as:

- **Mu (μ):** mediates analgesia, euphoria, respiratory depression, and physical dependence.
- **Delta (δ):** contributes to spinal analgesia and mood modulation.
- **Kappa (κ):** associated with analgesia, dysphoria, and sedation.
- **Sigma (σ):** previously described but now excluded as it is not naloxone-reversible.

Modern nomenclature refers to:

- **MOP:** mu opioid peptide receptor.
- **DOP:** delta opioid peptide receptor.
- **KOP:** kappa opioid peptide receptor.
- **NOP:** nociceptin opioid peptide receptor (previously associated with σ).

Opioid drugs act as full agonists, partial agonists, antagonists, or mixed agonist–antagonists at these receptors, resulting in a wide range of clinical effects (Pasternak and Pan 2013; Stein 2016).

Clinical Uses

Opioids are used for:

- **Analgesia** in acute, chronic, and perioperative pain.
- **Adjuncts in anaesthesia** to blunt haemodynamic responses to surgical stimulation.
- **Palliative care,** providing relief of pain and breathlessness in advanced disease.
- **Suppression of cough** (e.g. codeine).
- **Treatment of diarrhoea** (e.g. loperamide).
- **Opioid substitution therapy** in dependence (e.g. methadone, buprenorphine) (Benyamin et al. 2008) (Table 4.2).

Table 4.2 Side effects of opioids

System	Effect
Respiratory	Respiratory depression (dose-dependent; primary cause of opioid-related deaths)
Gastrointestinal	Nausea, vomiting (via CTZ stimulation), constipation (due to reduced GI motility), delayed gastric emptying
Central nervous	Sedation, dizziness, confusion, euphoria or dysphoria, tolerance, dependence
Dermatological	Pruritus (especially face/neck/chest), often due to histamine release
Endocrine	Suppression of hypothalamic-pituitary axis with long-term use (↓ cortisol, ↓ testosterone)
Cardiovascular	Bradycardia, hypotension (especially with morphine, due to histamine release)

Tolerance, Dependence, and Addiction
Repeated opioid exposure leads to tolerance, in which increasing doses are needed to maintain effect. Tolerance develops to analgesic and euphoric effects but typically not to constipation or miosis. Dependence refers to physiological adaptation, such that abrupt discontinuation precipitates a withdrawal syndrome characterised by rhinorrhoea, lacrimation, yawning, restlessness, nausea, vomiting, diarrhoea, tachycardia, hypertension, mydriasis, and piloerection ("cold turkey"). Addiction is distinct, describing compulsive use despite harm, and reflects psychological and behavioural components (Kosten and George 2002).

Histamine Release
Natural opioids such as morphine and codeine may cause histamine release, producing pruritus, flushing, and hypotension. These effects can be attenuated by antihistamines such as chlorphenamine or diphenhydramine. Synthetic opioids, including fentanyl and remifentanil, are less likely to provoke histamine release (Smith and Elliott 2012) (Table 4.3).

4.2.1 Morphine

Uses
Morphine is a potent opioid analgesic used in the management of moderate-to-severe pain, both acute (e.g. trauma, perioperative) and chronic (e.g. cancer, palliative care). It is also employed in acute myocardial infarction to relieve anxiety and reduce cardiac preload and afterload through vasodilation. In pulmonary oedema and congestive cardiac failure, morphine improves ventilation–perfusion matching and alleviates dyspnoea. Additionally, it is used in labour analgesia and via spinal or epidural routes for postoperative and obstetric analgesia (Hanna and Peat 2014).

Mechanism of Action
Morphine is an agonist at μ-opioid (MOP) and κ-opioid (KOP) receptors, which are G-protein–coupled receptors linked to Gi/o proteins. Activation inhibits adenylyl cyclase, reducing cyclic AMP, opens potassium channels to hyperpolarise neurons, and inhibits calcium influx, thereby reducing presynaptic neurotransmitter release (e.g. substance P, glutamate). The net effect is attenuation of nociceptive transmission at spinal and supraspinal levels (Pasternak 2010).

Table 4.3 Opioid potency comparison

Drug	Relative potency
Morphine	1×
Hydromorphone	10×
Fentanyl	100×
Remifentanil	250×
Sufentanil	Up to 1000×

Pharmacokinetics

Morphine can be administered by various routes, including oral, sublingual, rectal, inhaled, subcutaneous, intramuscular, intravenous, epidural, and intrathecal. Oral bioavailability is low (~30%) due to first-pass metabolism, while rectal administration achieves ~50% bioavailability. Morphine exhibits low protein binding (~30%) and is metabolised in the liver by UGT enzymes to morphine-3-glucuronide (M3G, inactive and potentially neurotoxic at high levels) and morphine-6-glucuronide (M6G, active with greater potency than morphine). Elimination is predominantly renal (~90%), with a half-life of 2–4 h, prolonged in renal impairment due to M6G accumulation (Osborne et al. 1990).

Adverse Effects

Morphine produces systemic, dose-dependent side effects:

- **Cardiovascular:** mild hypotension and bradycardia (via vagal stimulation); histamine release contributing to vasodilation.
- **Respiratory:** dose-dependent respiratory depression by suppressing brainstem responses to CO_2 and hypoxia.
- **Neurological:** sedation, euphoria, dizziness, tolerance, and physical dependence.
- **Gastrointestinal:** constipation from myenteric plexus inhibition; nausea and vomiting via the chemoreceptor trigger zone and delayed gastric emptying.
- **Genitourinary:** urinary retention due to increased sphincter tone.
- **Endocrine:** suppression of ACTH, LH, and FSH, leading to reduced libido and menstrual irregularities.
- **Immunological:** histamine-mediated pruritus, urticaria, and bronchospasm (Hanna and Peat 2014).

Other Considerations

Accumulation of M6G in renal failure can cause prolonged sedation and respiratory depression, necessitating dose adjustment. Morphine should be used cautiously with other CNS depressants such as benzodiazepines. Cross-tolerance with other opioids occurs but is often incomplete. Morphine has significant abuse potential due to its euphoric effects (Osborne et al. 1990).

Typical Dosing

- **Intrathecal:** 100–500 micrograms (profound, long-lasting effect).
- **Epidural:** 1–5 mg for obstetric or major surgical analgesia.
- **Intravenous:** 0.05–0.1 mg/kg every 2–3 h, titrated to effect.
- **Intramuscular/subcutaneous:** 0.1–0.2 mg/kg every 2–3 h.
- **Oral:** 10–30 mg every 4 h, with slow-release formulations used for chronic pain (Hanna and Peat 2014).

4.2.2 Fentanyl

Uses

Fentanyl is a synthetic opioid widely used for its potent analgesic and sedative properties. In anaesthesia, it is used during induction to blunt the sympathetic response to laryngoscopy and intubation, and for maintenance of intraoperative analgesia. It is also employed for postoperative pain control, chronic pain management (notably in palliative care via transdermal patches), and as an adjunct to neuraxial anaesthesia via epidural or intrathecal routes. Rapid-onset formulations, such as buccal, sublingual, and intranasal, are used for breakthrough cancer pain. Fentanyl is also a component of procedural sedation, often in combination with benzodiazepines (Stanley 2014; Prommer 2009).

Mechanism of Action

Fentanyl is a highly selective μ-opioid (MOP) receptor agonist. By inhibiting ascending pain pathways and altering the perception and emotional response to pain, it produces profound analgesia, sedation, and euphoria (Prommer 2009).

Pharmacokinetics

Fentanyl is approximately 100 times more potent than morphine, largely due to its extreme lipid solubility, which allows rapid penetration of the central nervous system and fast onset of action. It is highly protein bound (~85%) and metabolised hepatically by CYP3A4 to inactive metabolites. Routes of administration include intravenous (IV), intramuscular (IM), epidural, intrathecal, transdermal, buccal, sublingual, and intranasal. Elimination occurs primarily via renal excretion. The pharmacokinetics vary by route:

- **IV distribution half-life:** ~6–8 min.
- **Transdermal half-life:** ~17 h.
- **Intrathecal duration:** up to 16 h due to cerebrospinal fluid depot effect (Prommer 2009; Stanley 2014).

Adverse Effects

Fentanyl shares the typical opioid side-effect profile, with some unique features:

- **Cardiovascular:** bradycardia (via vagal stimulation), mild hypotension with minimal histamine release.
- **Respiratory:** profound dose-dependent respiratory depression, reduced ventilatory response to CO_2 and hypoxia, and chest wall rigidity with high or rapid IV doses (Dahan et al. 2010).
- **Gastrointestinal:** nausea, vomiting, and constipation.
- **Genitourinary:** urinary retention.

- **Endocrine:** suppression of hypothalamic–pituitary axis, reduced libido, and testosterone suppression with chronic use.
- **Neurological:** sedation, dizziness, euphoria, dependence, tolerance, and addiction risk (Prommer 2009).

Other Considerations

Fentanyl has a rapid onset (<60 seconds IV; 5–10 min transdermal) and short duration of action (20–40 min after IV bolus), though longer with transdermal application. Transdermal patches should be used cautiously, as heat, fever, or damaged skin can increase absorption and risk of toxicity. Fentanyl has high abuse potential and is frequently implicated in synthetic opioid-related overdose deaths. Its versatility and high potency make it a common choice in opioid rotation protocols (Stanley 2014; Prommer 2009).

Typical Dosing

- **IV analgesia:** 25–50 micrograms every 5–10 min as needed.
- **IV induction:** 100–200 micrograms prior to laryngoscopy.
- **Epidural adjunct:** 25–100 micrograms combined with local anaesthetic.
- **Intrathecal adjunct:** 10–25 micrograms as part of spinal anaesthesia.
- **Transdermal patch:** 12–100 micrograms/hour, replaced every 72 h.
- **Buccal/intranasal:** 100–400 micrograms for breakthrough cancer pain

4.2.3 Remifentanyl

Uses

Remifentanil is an ultra–short-acting synthetic opioid used primarily for intraoperative analgesia as part of balanced anaesthesia. It is also employed in patient-controlled analgesia (PCA) for labour analgesia in patients for whom neuraxial techniques are contraindicated, such as those on anticoagulation. Other indications include sedation and analgesia in critically ill, ventilated patients, and as an adjunct for controlled hypotensive anaesthesia during neurosurgical or ENT procedures (Sneyd and Rigby-Jones 2010).

Mechanism of Action

Remifentanil is a potent μ-opioid receptor (MOP) agonist. Activation of the receptor inhibits adenylyl cyclase, opens potassium channels (causing hyperpolarisation), and closes voltage-gated calcium channels, thereby reducing neurotransmitter release. These actions result in profound analgesia, sedation, and suppression of sympathetic tone (Egan 1995).

Pharmacokinetics
Remifentanil is administered exclusively by intravenous infusion or bolus, as it is unsuitable for oral use due to rapid metabolism. It is approximately 100–200 times more potent than morphine and about twice as potent as fentanyl. Its metabolism is unique among opioids, relying on rapid hydrolysis by non-specific plasma and tissue esterases, independent of hepatic or renal function, making it ideal for patients with organ impairment. Remifentanil has a low volume of distribution and minimal tissue accumulation. The elimination half-life is approximately 3–10 min, and its context-sensitive half-time remains short (~3–5 min) even after prolonged infusions, making it particularly suited for total intravenous anaesthesia (TIVA) (Glass et al. 1993; Egan 1995).

Adverse Effects
Remifentanil's side effects are typical of potent opioids:

- **Cardiovascular:** bradycardia and hypotension from reduced sympathetic tone.
- **Respiratory:** profound dose-dependent respiratory depression.
- **Neuromuscular:** generalised muscle rigidity, particularly with rapid bolus administration.
- **Other:** nausea, vomiting, euphoria, dizziness, urinary retention, and occasionally pruritus.

Due to its very short duration of action, pain may return abruptly at the end of the infusion; a longer-acting analgesic should be administered preemptively (Sneyd and Rigby-Jones 2010).

Precautions
Remifentanil should not be used as the sole agent for postoperative analgesia, as its effects dissipate quickly. It is contraindicated in patients with known hypersensitivity to fentanyl analogues. Rapid bolus administration should be avoided due to the risk of chest wall rigidity and apnoea (Glass et al. 1993).

Dosage
- **Infusion:** 0.05–2 micrograms/kg/min, typically titrated within the range of 0.1–0.5 micrograms/kg/min.
- **Bolus:** not routinely recommended, but if used, doses <0.5 micrograms/kg should be given slowly (Egan 1995).

4.2.4 Tramadol

Uses

Tramadol is a centrally acting analgesic indicated for the management of moderate to moderately severe acute pain. It may also be used for selected cases of chronic pain, particularly when conventional opioids are unsuitable. Tramadol is frequently combined with paracetamol or NSAIDs as part of a multimodal analgesia strategy (Leppert 2009).

Mechanism of Action

Tramadol has a unique multimodal mechanism of action. It is a weak agonist at μ-opioid (MOP) receptors, with minor activity at κ (KOP) and δ (DOP) receptors. It also inhibits the reuptake of noradrenaline and serotonin, enhancing descending inhibitory pain pathways, and stimulates central serotonin release. The active metabolite, O-desmethyltramadol, produced via hepatic metabolism, has a higher affinity for MOP receptors and accounts for much of the opioid effect (Grond and Sablotzki 2004; Trescot et al. 2008).

Pharmacokinetics

Tramadol is administered orally, intravenously, intramuscularly, or rectally. Oral bioavailability is approximately 75% and increases with repeated dosing due to reduced first-pass metabolism. It is minimally protein bound (~20%) and metabolised in the liver by CYP2D6 and CYP3A4 to form O-desmethyltramadol (active) and N-desmethyltramadol (inactive). CYP2D6 genetic polymorphisms influence metabolism, with poor or ultra-rapid metabolisers showing altered efficacy and risk. Tramadol and its metabolites are primarily excreted renally, and dose adjustment is required in renal impairment. The elimination half-life is about 6 h but may be prolonged in hepatic or renal dysfunction. Tramadol is approximately one-tenth as potent as morphine (Grond and Sablotzki 2004).

Adverse Effects

Tramadol is associated with the following side effects:

- **Common:** nausea, vomiting (more frequent than with morphine), constipation, dizziness, headache, and sedation.
- **Cardiovascular:** mild hypotension and bradycardia.
- **Respiratory:** dose-dependent respiratory depression, typically less severe than morphine.
- **Neuropsychiatric:** lowers seizure threshold—contraindicated in epilepsy—and may precipitate serotonin syndrome when combined with SSRIs, MAOIs, or other serotonergic agents.
- **Endocrine:** suppression of the hypothalamic–pituitary–gonadal axis, potentially reducing libido and mood.
- **Genitourinary:** urinary retention from increased sphincter tone.

- **Dermatologic:** rash, pruritus, and urticaria due to histamine release (Leppert 2009; Trescot et al. 2008).

Precautions and Contraindications

Tramadol is contraindicated in children under 12 years, in patients under 18 years after tonsillectomy or adenoidectomy, and during pregnancy or lactation due to risks of neonatal withdrawal and respiratory depression. It is also contraindicated in patients with seizure disorders or those taking serotonergic drugs due to the risk of serotonin syndrome. Caution is advised in elderly patients and those with renal or hepatic impairment (Grond and Sablotzki 2004).

Dosage

- **Oral:** 50–100 mg every 6 h as needed.
- **Maximum daily dose:** 400 mg in adults, reduced in elderly or patients with renal or hepatic dysfunction (Leppert 2009).

4.2.5 Codeine

Uses

Codeine is a weak opioid used for the management of mild-to-moderate pain, typically in combination with paracetamol or NSAIDs as part of a multimodal analgesia strategy. It is also used as an antitussive to suppress the cough reflex and occasionally as an antidiarrhoeal agent, particularly in irritable bowel syndrome and chronic diarrhoea (Trescot et al. 2008).

Mechanism of Action

Codeine itself is a weak agonist at μ-opioid (MOP), δ-opioid (DOP), κ-opioid (KOP), and nociceptin (NOP) receptors. It acts largely as a prodrug, with approximately 5–10% of an administered dose metabolised in the liver by CYP2D6 to morphine, which provides the principal analgesic effect through MOP receptor activation. Other metabolites include norcodeine (inactive) and codeine-6-glucuronide (minimally active) (Lotsch et al. 2009; Trescot et al. 2008).

Pharmacokinetics

Codeine is well absorbed after oral, rectal, subcutaneous, or intramuscular administration, with oral bioavailability of approximately 90%. It undergoes extensive first-pass hepatic metabolism via CYP2D6, CYP3A4, and glucuronidation. Codeine and its metabolites are excreted primarily in the urine. Protein binding is low (~10%), and the elimination half-life is around 3 h (Lotsch et al. 2009).

Adverse Effects

- **Central nervous system:** sedation, dizziness, euphoria, and headache.
- **Respiratory:** dose-dependent respiratory depression, with reduced sensitivity to hypercapnia and hypoxia.
- **Gastrointestinal:** constipation from decreased peristalsis, and nausea and vomiting from chemoreceptor trigger zone stimulation.
- **Cardiovascular:** orthostatic hypotension, particularly in elderly or hypovolaemic patients.
- **Genitourinary:** urinary retention.
- **Other:** pruritus, sweating, and dependence with chronic use (Trescot et al. 2008).

Other Considerations

Codeine metabolism is subject to genetic variability in CYP2D6 activity. Approximately 10% of Caucasians are poor metabolisers and derive little analgesia, whereas 1–2% are ultra-rapid metabolisers, producing excessive morphine and at increased risk of toxicity. Codeine is contraindicated in children under 12 years, in patients undergoing tonsillectomy or adenoidectomy, and in breastfeeding mothers due to the risk of severe respiratory depression and death (Kelly et al. 2012). Caution is required when combining codeine with other CNS depressants or serotonergic agents.

Dosage

- **Adults:** 30–60 mg orally every 4–6 h as needed, with a maximum daily dose of 240 mg.
- **Children:** use is generally avoided due to safety concerns; historically, doses of 1 mg/kg every 6 h were used but are now discouraged (Kelly et al. 2012).

Conflicts of Interest The authors have no conflicts of interest to declare that are relevant to the content of this chapter.

References

Antithrombotic Trialists' Collaboration (2002) 'Collaborative meta-analysis of randomised trials of antiplatelet therapy for prevention of death, myocardial infarction, and stroke in high-risk patients', *BMJ*, 324(7329), pp. 71–86.

Benyamin, R., Trescot, A.M., Datta, S., Buenaventura, R., Adlaka, R., Sehgal, N., Glaser, S.E. and Vallejo, R. (2008) 'Opioid complications and side effects', *Pain Physician*, 11(2 Suppl), pp. S105–S120.

Bombardier, C., Laine, L., Reicin, A., Shapiro, D., Burgos-Vargas, R., Davis, B., Day, R., Ferraz, M.B., Hawkey, C.J., Hochberg, M.C., Kvien, T.K. and Schnitzer, T.J. (2000) 'Comparison of upper gastrointestinal toxicity of rofecoxib and naproxen in patients with rheumatoid arthritis', *New England Journal of Medicine*, 343(21), pp. 1520–1528.

Dahan, A., Aarts, L. and Smith, T.W. (2010) 'Incidence, reversal, and prevention of opioid-induced respiratory depression', *Anesthesiology*, 112(1), pp. 226–238.

Egan, T.D. (1995) 'Remifentanil pharmacokinetics and pharmacodynamics. A preliminary appraisal', *Clinical Pharmacokinetics*, 29(2), pp. 80–94.

Forrest, J.A.H., Clements, J.A. and Prescott, L.F. (1982) 'Clinical pharmacokinetics of paracetamol', *Clinical Pharmacokinetics*, 7(2), pp. 93–107.

Glass, P.S., Hardman, D., Kamiyama, Y., Quill, T.J., Marton, G., Donn, K.H., Grosse, C.M. and Hermann, D.J. (1993) 'Preliminary pharmacokinetics and pharmacodynamics of an ultra-short-acting opioid: remifentanil (GI87084B)', *Anesth Analg*, 77(6), pp. 1031–1040.

Graham, G.G. and Scott, K.F. (2005) 'Mechanism of action of paracetamol', *American Journal of Therapeutics*, 12(1), pp. 46–55.

Grosser, T., Fries, S. and FitzGerald, G.A. (2006) 'Biological basis for the cardiovascular consequences of COX-2 inhibition: therapeutic challenges and opportunities', *Journal of Clinical Investigation*, 116(1), pp. 4–15.

Grosser, T., Smyth, E. and FitzGerald, G.A. (2017) 'Anti-inflammatory, antipyretic, and analgesic agents; pharmacotherapy of gout', in Brunton, L.L., Hilal-Dandan, R. and Knollmann, B.C. (eds.) *Goodman & Gilman's The Pharmacological Basis of Therapeutics*. 13th edn. New York: McGraw-Hill, pp. 671–716.

Grond, S. and Sablotzki, A. (2004) 'Clinical pharmacology of tramadol', *Clinical Pharmacokinetics*, 43(13), pp. 879–923.

Hanna, M. and Peat, S. (2014) 'Morphine in cancer pain: current status and future directions', *Expert Review of Clinical Pharmacology*, 7(6), pp. 777–785.

Heard, K.J. (2008) 'Acetylcysteine for acetaminophen poisoning', *New England Journal of Medicine*, 359(3), pp. 285–292.

Kelly, L.E., Rieder, M., van den Anker, J., Malkin, B., Ross, C.J.D., Neely, M.N., Carleton, B. and Hayden, M.R. (2012) 'More codeine fatalities after tonsillectomy in North American children', *Pediatrics*, 129(5), pp. e1343–e1347.

Kosten, T.R. and George, T.P. (2002) 'The neurobiology of opioid dependence: implications for treatment', *Science & Practice Perspectives*, 1(1), pp. 13–20.

Leppert, W. (2009) 'Tramadol as an analgesic for mild to moderate cancer pain', *Pharmacological Reports*, 61(6), pp. 978–992.

Lotsch, J., Geisslinger, G. and Tegeder, I. (2009) 'Pharmacokinetics of opioids in liver disease', *Clinical Pharmacokinetics*, 48(3), pp. 155–168.

Moncada, S. and Vane, J.R. (1979) 'Pharmacology and endogenous roles of prostaglandin endoperoxides, thromboxane A2, and prostacyclin', *Pharmacological Reviews*, 30(3), pp. 293–331.

Osborne, R., Joel, S., Trew, D. and Slevin, M. (1990) 'Morphine and metabolites: characteristics and clinical implications', *British Journal of Clinical Pharmacology*, 30(5), pp. 514–524.

Pasternak, G.W. (2010) 'Molecular insights into μ opioid pharmacology: from the clinic to the bench', *Clinical Journal of Pain*, 26(Suppl 10), pp. S3–S9.

Pasternak, G.W. and Pan, Y.X. (2013) 'Mu opioids and their receptors: evolution of a concept', *Pharmacological Reviews*, 65(4), pp. 1257–1317.

Patrono, C., García Rodríguez, L.A., Landolfi, R. and Baigent, C. (2005) 'Low-dose aspirin for the prevention of atherothrombosis', *New England Journal of Medicine*, 353(22), pp. 2373–2383.

Patrono, C., Morais, J., Baigent, C., Collet, J.P., Fitzgerald, D., Halvorsen, S., Rocca, B., Siegbahn, A. and Storey, R.F. (2017) 'Antiplatelet agents for the treatment and prevention of coronary atherothrombosis', *Journal of the American College of Cardiology*, 70(16), pp. 1991–2010.

Prescott, L.F. (2000) 'Paracetamol: past, present, and future', *American Journal of Therapeutics*, 7(2), pp. 143–147.

Proudfoot, A.T. and Krenzelok, E.P. (2010) 'Aspirin (acetylsalicylic acid) poisoning', *Clinical Toxicology*, 48(5), pp. 456–457.

Prommer, E. (2009) 'Fentanyl: a pharmacological review', *Cancer*, 115(9), pp. 2009–2021.

Rumack, B.H. (2002) 'Acetaminophen misconceptions', *Hepatology*, 36(4 Pt 1), pp. 983–984.

Smith, H.S. and Elliott, J.A. (2012) 'Opioid-induced histamine release and its clinical relevance', *Pain Physician*, 15(3), pp. 237–248.

Sneyd, J.R. and Rigby-Jones, A.E. (2010) 'Remifentanil and anaesthesia', *Anaesthesia*, 65(s1), pp. 45–54.
Stanley, T.H. (2014) 'The fentanyl story', *Journal of Pain*, 15(12), pp. 1215–1226.
Stein, C. (2016) 'Opioid receptors', *Annual Review of Medicine*, 67, pp. 433–451.
Trescot, A.M., Datta, S., Lee, M. and Hansen, H. (2008) 'Opioid pharmacology', *Pain Physician*, 11(2 Suppl), pp. S133–S153.
Vane, J.R. and Botting, R.M. (1995) 'New insights into the mode of action of anti-inflammatory drugs', *Inflammation Research*, 44(1), pp. 1–10.
Vane, J.R. and Botting, R.M. (1998) 'Mechanism of action of anti-inflammatory drugs', *International Journal of Tissue Reactions*, 20(1–2), pp. 3–15.
Vane, J.R. and Botting, R.M. (2003) 'The mechanism of action of aspirin', *Thrombosis Research*, 110(5–6), pp. 255–258.
Warner, T.D. and Mitchell, J.A. (2004) 'Cyclooxygenase-3 (COX-3): filling in the gaps toward a COX continuum?', *Proceedings of the National Academy of Sciences of the United States of America*, 101(34), pp. 12469–12470.

Antiemetic Drugs

5

5.1 Antiemetic Drugs

Antiemetics are a diverse group of drugs used to prevent and treat nausea and vomiting (N + V), which are common symptoms across many clinical contexts. Indications include postoperative nausea and vomiting (PONV), motion sickness, chemotherapy-induced nausea and vomiting (CINV), radiotherapy, hyperemesis gravidarum, and medication-induced nausea (e.g. from opioids) (Shaikh et al. 2016). Effective antiemetic therapy depends on an understanding of the neurophysiological pathways underpinning the emetic reflex, which is coordinated by brainstem nuclei collectively termed the vomiting centre. This centre integrates input from several afferent pathways (Denholm and Gallaghe 2018).

Physiology of Nausea and Vomiting

The vomiting centre, located in the medulla oblongata, serves as the final common pathway for the emetic reflex. It receives inputs from multiple sources:

- Chemoreceptor trigger zone (CTZ): located in the area postrema, outside the blood–brain barrier, sensitive to blood-borne emetogens such as opioids, uraemic toxins, and chemotherapeutic agents. Key receptors include dopamine D_2, serotonin 5-HT_3, neurokinin NK_1, and opioid receptors.
- Gastrointestinal tract and vagal afferents: activated by distension, irritation, toxins, or cytotoxic drugs, mediated via 5-HT_3 and D_2 receptors.
- Vestibular system: important in motion sickness and vestibular disorders, mediated through histamine H_1 and muscarinic M_1 receptors.
- Higher cortical centres: respond to psychological stimuli such as fear, pain, or anticipation, involving H_1 and M_1 receptors.
- Baroreceptors and chemoreceptors: activated by hypotension, hypoxia, and other metabolic derangements, signalling via vagal afferents to the brainstem (Singla and Singh 2016; Denholm and Gallaghe 2018).

G. Browne, *PharmacologyPro*, https://doi.org/10.1007/978-3-032-10227-0_5

Multimodal Antiemetic Strategy

No single antiemetic is fully effective in all patients or settings. Combining drugs from different classes, each targeting a distinct pathway, improves efficacy and minimises side effects. For example, the combination of ondansetron and dexamethasone is widely used in surgical patients, and in high-risk scenarios, adding a dopamine antagonist or NK_1 antagonist further enhances protection (Shaikh et al. 2016).

Special Considerations

Several safety and tolerability issues are important when selecting antiemetics:

- QT prolongation: drugs such as ondansetron and droperidol can prolong the QT interval and should be used with caution in patients with cardiac risk factors.
- Extrapyramidal side effects (EPSEs): dopamine antagonists (e.g. metoclopramide, prochlorperazine) may cause dystonia, akathisia, and Parkinsonian symptoms, especially in younger patients.
- Sedation: common with antihistamines and antipsychotics, which may be undesirable in some contexts.
- Pregnancy: cyclizine and ondansetron are generally considered safe, particularly in the second and third trimesters (Singla and Singh 2016; Shaikh et al. 2016) (Table 5.1).

Table 5.1 Classes of antiemetic drugs

Drug class	Example(s)	Mechanism of action	Common indications
5-HT3 Antagonists	Ondansetron, Granisetron	Block 5-HT3 receptors in CTZ and GI tract	PONV, CINV
D2 Antagonists	Metoclopramide, Domperidone, Prochlorperazine, Haloperidol	Block dopamine D2 receptors in CTZ	PONV, gastroparesis, migraine-related N+V
Antihistamines (H1)	Cyclizine, Promethazine	Block H1 receptors in vestibular and cortical areas	Motion sickness, vertigo
Anticholinergics (M1)	Hyoscine (Scopolamine)	Block muscarinic receptors in vestibular system	Motion sickness
Steroids	Dexamethasone	Unclear; may reduce inflammation and serotonin release in the gut	CINV, PONV (especially in combination)
NK1 Antagonists	Aprepitant, Fosaprepitant	Block Substance P at NK1 receptors in CTZ	CINV, highly emetogenic chemotherapy
Cannabinoids	Nabilone, Dronabinol	Stimulate CB1 receptors in CNS	Refractory CINV, palliative care

5.2 Domperidone

Uses

Domperidone is a dopamine receptor antagonist used primarily for the management of nausea and vomiting, particularly in the context of delayed gastric emptying, functional dyspepsia, or secondary to medications such as opioids or levodopa. It also acts as a prokinetic agent, enhancing gastric motility in gastroesophageal reflux disease (GERD) and gastroparesis (Boyce 2011). Off-label, it may be used as a galactagogue to stimulate lactation by increasing prolactin secretion.

Mechanism of Action

Domperidone is a peripheral dopamine D_2 receptor antagonist with limited central nervous system penetration. Its antiemetic effect is mediated by D_2 blockade in the chemoreceptor trigger zone (CTZ), located outside the blood–brain barrier. In the gastrointestinal tract, D_2 antagonism promotes acetylcholine release, improving gastric emptying and motility. Compared to metoclopramide, domperidone is less likely to cause extrapyramidal side effects due to its poor CNS penetration (Chang 2010).

Pharmacokinetics

- Routes: Oral, intramuscular, rectal
- Oral bioavailability: ~15% (extensive first-pass metabolism); ~90% IM (Boyce 2011)
- Protein binding: >90%
- Metabolism: Hepatic and intestinal via CYP3A4 (Chang 2010)
- Half-life: ~7 h
- Excretion: Primarily faecal (via biliary excretion)

Adverse Effects

- Endocrine: Hyperprolactinaemia (galactorrhoea, gynaecomastia, amenorrhoea)
- Gastrointestinal: Abdominal cramps, diarrhoea, nausea
- Dermatological: Rash, urticaria, pruritus
- Cardiovascular: QT prolongation and rare ventricular arrhythmias, especially in predisposed individuals (Field et al. 2019; van Noord et al. 2010)
- Neurological: Drowsiness (uncommon); extrapyramidal side effects are rare (van Harten et al. 1999)

Other Considerations

The use of this drug carries important safety considerations. It should be avoided in patients with known QT prolongation, electrolyte abnormalities such as hypokalaemia, or those taking concurrent QT-prolonging agents, including amiodarone or fluconazole (Field et al. 2019). In addition, concomitant administration with strong CYP3A4 inhibitors, such as clarithromycin or ketoconazole, can increase the risk of cardiotoxicity (Chang 2010). Overall, the safety profile limits its recommendation for long-term use and in high-risk populations, particularly elderly patients with underlying cardiac disease (EMA 2014).

Dose
- Oral: 10 mg up to three times daily, taken 15–30 min before meals
- Intramuscular: 12.5 mg (used infrequently)
- Rectal: 30 mg suppository (for patients unable to take oral medications)

5.3 Prochlorperazine

Uses
Prochlorperazine is a phenothiazine derivative used primarily for its antiemetic properties. It is effective in treating nausea and vomiting from a range of causes, including postoperative nausea, chemotherapy-induced nausea, motion sickness, and migraine-associated nausea (Din 2023). It is also used in the management of vertigo due to vestibular disorders such as labyrinthitis and Ménière's disease. While originally developed as an antipsychotic, its use in psychiatric settings has largely been replaced by newer atypical agents.

Mechanism of Action
Prochlorperazine acts predominantly as a dopamine D_2 receptor antagonist within the chemoreceptor trigger zone (CTZ) and the central nervous system. It also possesses weak anticholinergic and alpha-adrenergic blocking activity, which contributes to both its therapeutic effects and side effect profile (Din 2023).

Pharmacokinetics
It may be administered orally, rectally, intramuscularly (IM), or intravenously (IV). Oral bioavailability is low (~12.5%) due to extensive first-pass hepatic metabolism (Isah 1991). Prochlorperazine is highly protein-bound (~99%) and undergoes extensive hepatic metabolism to inactive metabolites, which are eliminated via the biliary system and excreted in the faeces. The elimination half-life is approximately 6–8 h (Taylor 1987; Isah 1991).

Adverse Effects
Neurological side effects include extrapyramidal symptoms (EPSEs) such as acute dystonia, akathisia, Parkinsonism, and—more rarely—tardive dyskinesia and neuroleptic malignant syndrome (NMS), which is potentially life-threatening (Din 2023). Sedation and drowsiness are common, especially in older adults. Cardiovascular effects include orthostatic hypotension, particularly following IM or IV administration (Isah 1991). Its anticholinergic actions may lead to dry mouth, blurred vision, and urinary retention. Raised prolactin levels can result in galactorrhoea, gynaecomastia, and menstrual disturbances. Rare cases of cholestatic jaundice have been reported (Din 2023).

Other Considerations
Caution is advised in elderly patients due to the increased risk of EPSEs and postural hypotension. Prochlorperazine should be avoided in individuals with Parkinson's disease, as it may exacerbate motor symptoms. Although primarily used as an antiemetic, it shares class-related side effects with antipsychotic medications (Din 2023).

Dosing
Typical oral dosing is 5–20 mg, up to three times daily in divided doses. For intramuscular administration, 12.5 mg every 8 h may be used. Rectal suppositories are dosed at 25 mg twice daily. Intravenous use is uncommon due to the heightened risk of hypotension and extrapyramidal reactions and should be undertaken with caution (Isah 1991; Taylor 1987).

5.4 Metoclopramide

Uses
Metoclopramide is a centrally and peripherally acting antiemetic and prokinetic agent. It is commonly used to treat nausea and vomiting from a variety of causes, including postoperative states, chemotherapy, opioid use, and gastroparesis (Albibi and McCallum 1983). In gastrointestinal disorders such as reflux and functional dyspepsia, it improves gastric emptying and alleviates symptoms (Heckroth et al. 2021). It is frequently combined with analgesics in the management of acute migraine to enhance drug absorption and control nausea. Though occasionally used off-label as a galactagogue to stimulate prolactin release, this is not routinely recommended (Kalas et al. 2023).

Mechanism of Action
Metoclopramide's primary effect is through dopamine D_2 receptor antagonism at the chemoreceptor trigger zone (CTZ) and in the gastrointestinal tract. At higher doses, it also exhibits serotonin 5-HT_3 receptor antagonism, enhancing its antiemetic efficacy (Gralla and Herrstedt 2017). As a 5-HT_4 receptor agonist, it increases acetylcholine release in the enteric nervous system, thereby stimulating gastric motility. Weak muscarinic receptor activity further contributes to its prokinetic profile (Heckroth et al. 2021; Kalas et al. 2023).

Pharmacokinetics
Administered orally, intramuscularly, or intravenously, metoclopramide has good oral bioavailability (~80%) and low protein binding (~30%). It undergoes hepatic metabolism to inactive compounds and is excreted renally. The elimination half-life is approximately 6 h, though this may be prolonged in renal impairment (Heckroth et al. 2021).

Adverse Effects

Extrapyramidal side effects (EPSEs) are the most significant concern, particularly in young adults and the elderly. These include acute dystonia, oculogyric crisis, akathisia, Parkinsonian symptoms, and—rarely with prolonged use—tardive dyskinesia (Junqueira et al. 2023). Metoclopramide can also cause hyperprolactinaemia, leading to galactorrhoea, amenorrhoea, and gynaecomastia. Sedation, dizziness, and fatigue are common central side effects. Neuroleptic malignant syndrome, while rare, is a serious potential complication. In the gastrointestinal system, it increases lower oesophageal sphincter tone, enhances gastric emptying, and reduces pyloric tone. It also carries a small risk of QT prolongation and arrhythmias, especially at high doses or when given intravenously (Kalas et al. 2023; Junqueira et al. 2023).

Other Considerations

Due to the risk of tardive dyskinesia, metoclopramide is generally limited to short-term use (≤5 days). It is contraindicated in patients with Parkinson's disease, phaeochromocytoma, epilepsy, bowel obstruction, or a history of EPSEs. Caution is advised in both paediatric and elderly populations due to heightened susceptibility to adverse neurological effects (Heckroth et al. 2021; Junqueira et al. 2023).

Dosing

The typical oral dose is 10 mg three times daily (maximum 30 mg/day). When administered intramuscularly or intravenously, 10 mg every 8 h is standard. IV doses should be given slowly over a minimum of 3 min to reduce the risk of adverse effects (Kalas et al. 2023).

5.5 Cyclizine

Uses

Cyclizine is a widely used antiemetic, particularly effective for motion sickness, postoperative nausea and vomiting (PONV), and opioid-induced nausea. It is also used for symptomatic relief in vestibular disorders such as Ménière's disease, and plays a key role in palliative care, particularly for nausea related to raised intracranial pressure or visceral disease (Schaefer et al. 2024; McNeill et al. 2023).

Mechanism of Action

Cyclizine is a centrally acting histamine H_1 receptor antagonist with additional anticholinergic (muscarinic receptor antagonist) properties. These dual actions target the vomiting centre and vestibular nuclei, making it especially effective in motion-related and vestibular nausea (Schaefer et al. 2024).

Pharmacokinetics

Cyclizine is administered orally, intravenously, or intramuscularly, with an onset of action approximately 30 min after administration and peak effect within 1–2 h.

Oral bioavailability is around 60%. It is metabolised hepatically to inactive compounds, with an elimination half-life of approximately 20 h. Excretion occurs primarily via the kidneys (Vella-Brincat et al. 2012).

Adverse Effects
Sedation, dizziness, and impaired coordination are the most common side effects, reflecting its ability to cross the blood–brain barrier. Anticholinergic effects such as dry mouth, blurred vision, urinary retention, and constipation are frequently observed, and particular caution is advised in patients with prostatic hypertrophy, narrow-angle glaucoma, or urinary outflow obstruction. Cardiovascular effects, including mild hypotension and tachycardia, may occur—especially with rapid IV administration. Paradoxical excitation may occasionally be seen, particularly in paediatric patients (Schaefer et al. 2024).

Other Considerations
Cyclizine is preferred in palliative care for nausea secondary to raised intracranial pressure or opioid use, and is associated with a longer duration of action and less sedation than older antihistamines. When administered intravenously, compatibility with other drugs (e.g. morphine) must be confirmed, as precipitation in the IV line may occur (McNeill et al. 2023).

Dosing
In adults, the typical dose is 50 mg orally, IV, or IM, up to three times daily (maximum 150 mg/day). In children aged 6–12 years, doses of 0.1 mg/kg up to a maximum of 25 mg may be given three times daily. Cyclizine is not routinely recommended in children under 6 years of age (Schaefer et al. 2024).

5.6 Ondansetron

Uses
Ondansetron is a first-line antiemetic used in the prevention and treatment of nausea and vomiting in a variety of clinical settings. It is particularly effective for postoperative nausea and vomiting (PONV), chemotherapy-induced nausea and vomiting (CINV), and nausea associated with radiotherapy (Griddine and Bush 2023; Singh et al. 2012). Its efficacy is greatest when nausea is primarily mediated by serotonin release, such as in acute emetogenic stimuli (Kohler 1991).

Mechanism of Action
Ondansetron is a selective 5-hydroxytryptamine-3 (5-HT_3) receptor antagonist. It acts both peripherally on vagal afferent fibres in the gastrointestinal tract and centrally within the chemoreceptor trigger zone (CTZ) of the medulla. Unlike other serotonin receptors, the 5-HT_3 receptor is a ligand-gated ion channel, making it a unique pharmacological target for antiemetic therapy (Kohler 1991; Griddine and Bush 2023).

Pharmacokinetics

Ondansetron is available via oral, sublingual, rectal, intravenous (IV), and intramuscular (IM) routes. Oral bioavailability is approximately 60% due to first-pass hepatic metabolism. It is 60–70% protein bound and undergoes extensive metabolism via CYP3A4, CYP1A2, and CYP2D6 isoenzymes. The elimination half-life ranges from 3 to 6 h. Excretion occurs through both renal and biliary pathways (Kohler 1991; Griddine and Bush 2023).

Adverse Effects

Headache is the most common side effect. QT interval prolongation may occur in a dose-dependent manner, especially at higher doses or in patients with predisposing risk factors, occasionally leading to Torsades de Pointes (Lee 2017). Other cardiovascular effects include bradycardia, particularly with rapid IV administration. Constipation, dizziness, fatigue, flushing, and transient visual disturbances have also been reported. Rarely, ototoxicity may occur with rapid IV infusion (Griddine and Bush 2023).

Other Considerations

Ondansetron should be used cautiously in patients with congenital long QT syndrome or those taking other QT-prolonging agents (e.g. amiodarone, methadone) (Lee 2017). As it is non-sedating, it pairs well with other antiemetics such as dexamethasone or cyclizine in multimodal regimens. It has no role in the treatment of motion sickness, as it lacks activity in the vestibular system (Griddine and Bush 2023).

Dosing

In adults, 4–8 mg can be administered orally or intravenously every 8–12 h, with a typical maximum daily dose of 16 mg. In children, the recommended dose is 100 micrograms/kg (up to a maximum of 4 mg per dose), repeated every 8 h if required (Griddine and Bush 2023).

5.7 Dexamethasone

Uses

Dexamethasone is a long-acting synthetic glucocorticoid widely used for its antiemetic, anti-inflammatory, and immunosuppressive properties. It is frequently administered as part of multimodal prophylaxis for postoperative nausea and vomiting (PONV) and in combination with other agents for chemotherapy-induced nausea and vomiting (CINV) (Bansal 2024; Najafzadeh et al. 2023). Additional indications include the management of cerebral oedema, asthma, anaphylaxis, septic shock, spinal cord compression, and adrenal insufficiency. In regional anaesthesia, dexamethasone is increasingly used as an adjuvant to peripheral nerve blocks to prolong analgesic duration (Albrecht et al. 2024).

Mechanism of Action

Dexamethasone binds to intracellular glucocorticoid receptors, altering gene transcription and downregulating pro-inflammatory cytokines such as IL-1, IL-6, and TNF-α. It has minimal mineralocorticoid activity. The antiemetic mechanism remains incompletely understood but likely involves inhibition of central prostaglandin synthesis, modulation of serotonin turnover, and effects on the nucleus tractus solitarius and chemoreceptor trigger zone (CTZ) (Bansal 2024).

Pharmacokinetics

The drug is well absorbed orally, with a bioavailability of approximately 80–90%. It is administered via oral, intravenous (IV), intramuscular (IM), or perineural routes. Following IV administration, onset of action occurs within 1–2 h. It is approximately 77% protein bound and undergoes hepatic metabolism via CYP3A4, with renal excretion of inactive metabolites. Dexamethasone has a long elimination half-life of 36–54 h, making it effective for extended symptom control with single-dose use (Bansal 2024; Najafzadeh et al. 2023).

Adverse Effects

Adverse effects are rare with single-dose use for PONV. With prolonged or repeated dosing, side effects may include:

- Endocrine and metabolic: Hyperglycaemia (can occur even after a single dose), fluid retention, and hypokalaemia.
- Neurological: Insomnia, agitation, or euphoria.
- Gastrointestinal: Gastritis and, rarely, peptic ulceration.
- Immunosuppression: Increased susceptibility to infection with chronic use.
- Other: Impaired wound healing, myopathy, and adrenal suppression with prolonged administration (Bansal 2024).

Other Considerations

Dexamethasone is valued in perioperative care for its long duration of antiemetic effect—often lasting up to 24 h after a single dose (Najafzadeh et al. 2023). It has no sedative or cardiovascular properties, making it an ideal adjunct in high-risk patients. However, caution is advised in diabetic patients due to potential glucose elevation, even after a single administration (Bansal 2024).

Dosing

- PONV prophylaxis: 4–8 mg IV at induction of anaesthesia (Najafzadeh et al. 2023; Ho et al. 2011)
- CINV: 8–20 mg IV depending on chemotherapy regimen (Bansal 2024)
- Peripheral nerve blocks: 4–10 mg perineurally to prolong block duration (off-label use) (Albrecht et al. 2024)

5.8 Aprepitant

Uses

Aprepitant is a selective neurokinin-1 (NK_1) receptor antagonist used for the prevention of nausea and vomiting (Diemunsch 2009). Its primary indication is in chemotherapy-induced nausea and vomiting (CINV), particularly with highly or moderately emetogenic regimens (Hesketh et al. 2003; Albany et al. 2012). It is also used for prophylaxis of postoperative nausea and vomiting (PONV), especially in high-risk patients or those unresponsive to conventional agents (Meyer et al. 2023). Aprepitant is commonly used as part of a multimodal antiemetic strategy alongside 5-HT_3 antagonists (e.g. ondansetron) and dexamethasone (Albany et al. 2012; Ibrahim 2024).

Mechanism of Action

Aprepitant blocks NK_1 receptors in the central nervous system, particularly in the nucleus tractus solitarius and area postrema, preventing binding of substance P—a key neuropeptide involved in the emetic reflex. While 5-HT_3 antagonists primarily control early-onset nausea, NK_1 antagonists are particularly effective at preventing delayed-phase vomiting (24–72 h post-chemotherapy) (Hesketh et al. 2003).

Pharmacokinetics

Aprepitant is administered orally, while its prodrug fosaprepitant is available for intravenous use. Oral bioavailability is approximately 60–65%, with extensive protein binding (>95%). It undergoes hepatic metabolism via CYP3A4, with minor contributions from CYP1A2 and CYP2C19. The elimination half-life is 9–13 h (longer for metabolites), and excretion is predominantly faecal via biliary routes (Hesketh et al. 2003; Albany et al. 2012).

Adverse Effects

Aprepitant is generally well tolerated. Common side effects include gastrointestinal disturbance (e.g. constipation, diarrhoea, anorexia), fatigue, dizziness, hiccups, and mild elevations in liver transaminases. Rare hypersensitivity reactions have been reported with intravenous fosaprepitant (Meyer et al. 2023).

Other Considerations

As a moderate inhibitor and inducer of CYP3A4, aprepitant may alter plasma levels of co-administered drugs. It increases concentrations of dexamethasone, midazolam, and other CYP3A4 substrates—dose adjustments may be necessary. It may also lower INR in patients on warfarin; close monitoring of coagulation is advised. Due to cost, its use is typically reserved for patients at high risk of emesis or those with prior prophylaxis failure. Data on use in pregnancy are limited (Meyer et al. 2023).

Dosing

- PONV prophylaxis: 40 mg orally, 1–3 h before anaesthesia (Meyer et al. 2023)
- CINV (3-day regimen):
  - Day 1: 125 mg orally, 1 h before chemotherapy
  - Days 2–3: 80 mg orally once daily (Hesketh et al. 2003; Albany et al. 2012)

References

Albany, C., Brames, M.J., Fausel, C., et al. (2012) 'Randomized, double-blind, placebo-controlled, phase III crossover study of aprepitant in combination with a 5-HT_3 antagonist and dexamethasone for cisplatin-induced nausea and vomiting', *Cancer Chemotherapy and Pharmacology*, 69(2), pp. 405–412.

Albrecht, E., Renard, Y. and Desai, N. (2024) 'Intravenous versus perineural dexamethasone to prolong analgesia after peripheral nerve blocks: systematic review with meta-analysis', *British Journal of Anaesthesia*, 133(1), pp. 59–72.

Albibi, R. and McCallum, R.W. (1983) 'Metoclopramide: pharmacology and clinical application', *Annals of Internal Medicine*, 98(1), pp. 86–93.

Bansal, T. (2024) 'Dexamethasone in anesthesia practice: a narrative review', *Journal of Anaesthesiology Clinical Pharmacology*, 40(1), pp. 1–7.

Boyce, M.J. (2011) 'Pharmacokinetic interaction between domperidone and ketoconazole', *Cancer Chemotherapy and Pharmacology*, 67(3), pp. 421–426.

Chang, S.Y. (2010) 'Mechanism-based inhibition of human cytochrome P450 3A by domperidone', *Biochemical Pharmacology*, 80(3), pp. 292–300.

Denholm, L. and Gallagher G. (2018) Physiology and pharmacology of nausea and vomiting. *Anaesthesia & Intensive Care Medicine*, 19(6), pp. 315–324. https://doi.org/10.1016/j.mpaic.2018.06.010.

Diemunsch, P. (2009) 'Neurokinin-1 receptor antagonists in the prevention of postoperative nausea and vomiting', *Current Opinion in Anesthesiology*, 22(6), pp. 713–719.

Din, L. (2023) 'Prochlorperazine', in *StatPearls* [Internet]. Treasure Island (FL): StatPearls Publishing. Available at: NCBI Bookshelf. [Accessed 1 September 2025].

EMA (2014) 'Domperidone-containing medicines: risk of cardiac side effects — restricted indication, contraindications and reduced dose'. European Medicines Agency Safety Review. [Online]. [Accessed 1 September 2025].

Field, J., Wasilewski, M., Bhuta, R., Malik, Z., Cooper, J., Parkman, H.P. and Schey, R. (2019) 'Effect of chronic domperidone use on QT interval', *Journal of Clinical Gastroenterology*, 53(9), pp. 648–652.

Gralla, R.J. and Herrstedt, J. (2017) 'Antiemetic agents: dopamine antagonists, antihistamines, and others', in Olver, I., Davis, H. and Hesketh, P.J. (eds.) *Supportive Care in Cancer: Antiemetic Therapy*. Cham: Springer, pp. 65–80.

Griddine, A. and Bush, K. (2023) 'Ondansetron', in *StatPearls* [Internet]. Treasure Island (FL): StatPearls Publishing. Available at: NCBI Bookshelf. [Accessed 1 September 2025].

Heckroth, M., et al. (2021) 'Nausea and vomiting in 2021: a comprehensive update', *Neurogastroenterology & Motility*, 33(4), e14022.

Hesketh, P.J., Grunberg, S.M., Gralla, R.J., Warr, D.G., Roila, F., de Wit, R., Chawla, S.P., Carides, A.D., Ianus, J., Elmer, M.E., Evans, J.K., Beck, K., Reines, S. and Horgan, K.J. (2003) Aprepitant Protocol 052 Study Group. The oral neurokinin-1 antagonistaprepitant for the prevention of chemotherapy-induced nausea and vomiting: a multinational, randomized, doubleblind,placebo-controlled trial in patients receiving high-dose cisplatin. *Journal of Clinical Oncology*, 21(22), pp. 4112–4119. https://doi.org/10.1200/JCO.2003.0[illegible].095.

Ho, C.M., Ho, S.T., Lee, T.Y. and Chiu, J.W. (2011) 'The optimal dose of prophylactic dexamethasone for postoperative nausea and vomiting: a meta-analysis of randomized controlled trials', *European Journal of Anaesthesiology*, 28(11), pp. 742–748.

Ibrahim, M.A. (2024) 'Antiemetic neurokinin-1 receptor blockers', in *StatPearls* [Internet]. Treasure Island (FL): StatPearls Publishing. Available at: https://www.ncbi.nlm.nih.gov/books/NBK470394/ [Accessed 1 September 2025].

Isah, A.O. (1991) 'Clinical pharmacology of prochlorperazine in healthy young males', *British Journal of Clinical Pharmacology*, 32(6), pp. 677–684.

Junqueira, D.R., et al. (2023) 'Restlessness and extrapyramidal events during metoclopramide treatment: a systematic review and meta-analysis', *Drugs in R&D*, 23(2), pp. 187–198.

Kalas, M.A., et al. (2023) 'Metoclopramide in gastroparesis: its mechanism of action and extrapyramidal side effects', *Gastrointestinal Disorders*, 5(3), p. 26.

Kohler, D.R. (1991) 'Ondansetron: a serotonin receptor (5-HT_3) antagonist for the prevention of nausea and vomiting', *Journal of Pharmacology and Experimental Therapeutics*, 256(1), pp. 363–370.

Lee, D.Y. (2017) 'Torsades de Pointes after ondansetron infusion in 2 patients', *Annals of Emergency Medicine*, 69(5), pp. 634–636.

McNeill, R., Donnelly, S., Laird, B.J. and Fallon, M. (2023) 'Cyclizine use in palliative care: a pharmacovigilance study', *BMJ Supportive & Palliative Care*, 13(e3), e1191.

Meyer, T.A., Habib, A.S., Wagner, D. and Gan, T.J. (2023) 'Neurokinin-1 receptor antagonists for the prevention of postoperative nausea and vomiting', *Pharmacotherapy*, 43(9), pp. 922–934.

Najafzadeh, M.J., Shafiei, M., Sharifi, M., Nazari, P., Nasiri, N. and Hashemian, M. (2023) 'The efficacy and safety of perioperative administration of dexamethasone: a systematic review and meta-analysis', *Ain-Shams Journal of Anesthesiology*, 15(1), p. 29.

Schaefer, T.S., Patel, P. and Zito, P.M. (2024) 'Antiemetic histamine H_1 receptor blockers', in *StatPearls* [Internet]. Treasure Island (FL): StatPearls Publishing. Available at: NCBI Bookshelf. [Accessed 1 September 2025].

Shaikh, S.I., Nagarekha, D., Hegade, G. and Marutheesh, M. (2016) 'Postoperative nausea and vomiting: a simple yet complex problem', *Anesthesia: Essays and Researches*, 10(3), pp. 388–396.

Singh, P., et al. (2012) 'Ondansetron: a review of pharmacokinetics and clinical experience in chemotherapy-induced nausea and vomiting', *Expert Opinion on Drug Metabolism & Toxicology*, 8(5), pp. 693–707.

Singla, P. and Singh, R. (2016) 'Nausea: a review of pathophysiology and therapeutics', *Therapeutic Advances in Gastroenterology*, 9(1), pp. 98–112.

Taylor, W.B. (1987) 'Preliminary studies of the pharmacokinetics of prochlorperazine', *British Journal of Clinical Pharmacology*, 23(2), pp. 137–142.

van Harten, P.N., Hoek, H.W. and Kahn, R.S. (1999) 'Acute dystonia induced by drug treatment', *BMJ*, 319(7210), pp. 623–626.

van Noord, C., Dieleman, J.P., van Herpen, G., Verhamme, K.M., Sturkenboom, M.C. and Stricker, B.H. (2010) 'Domperidone and ventricular arrhythmia or sudden cardiac death: a population-based case–control study in The Netherlands', *Drug Safety*, 33(11), pp. 1003–1014.

Vella-Brincat, J.W.A., Begg, E.J., Jensen, B.P., Chin, P.K.L., Roberts, R.L., Fairhall, M., MacLeod, S.A.D. and Reid, K. (2012) 'The pharmacokinetics and pharmacogenetics of the antiemetic cyclizine in palliative care patients', *Journal of Pain and Symptom Management*, 43(3), pp. 540–548.

6 Central Nervous System Drugs

6.1 Anticonvulsant Drugs

Anticonvulsants—also known as antiepileptic drugs (AEDs)—are primarily used in the prevention and treatment of epileptic seizures. Epilepsy is characterised by recurrent, unprovoked seizures caused by sudden, excessive, and synchronous neuronal discharges. These events may present as convulsions, sensory or behavioural changes, or altered consciousness. Beyond epilepsy, many anticonvulsants have broader clinical applications, including the management of neuropathic pain (e.g. trigeminal neuralgia, diabetic neuropathy), migraine prophylaxis, bipolar affective disorder (notably sodium valproate and lamotrigine), and as sedative agents in anaesthesia (e.g. benzodiazepines, barbiturates) (Wiffen et al. 2013).

Mechanisms of Action
AEDs stabilise neuronal activity through several key pathways:

- Inhibition of Voltage-Gated Sodium Channels: These agents prevent repetitive neuronal firing by stabilising sodium channels in their inactive state.
  Examples: phenytoin, carbamazepine, lamotrigine
- Enhancement of GABAergic Inhibition: GABA is the brain's principal inhibitory neurotransmitter. Drugs that increase GABA activity suppress neuronal excitability.
  Examples: benzodiazepines (e.g. midazolam), phenobarbital, sodium valproate
- Inhibition of T-Type Calcium Channels: These channels are implicated in thalamocortical rhythms, especially in absence seizures.
  Example: ethosuximide

G. Browne, *PharmacologyPro*, https://doi.org/10.1007/978-3-032-10227-0_6

- Inhibition of Glutamatergic Transmission: Some agents modulate glutamate release or receptor activity, reducing excitatory input.
  Examples: levetiracetam (via SV2A binding), perampanel (AMPA receptor antagonist).

Clinical Considerations

Perioperative Management

Maintenance of antiepileptic drug (AED) therapy in the perioperative period is essential to minimise the risk of seizures. Whenever possible, AEDs should be continued during fasting, with oral tablets taken alongside a small sip of water. If oral intake is not feasible, equivalent intravenous or rectal formulations should be used to ensure uninterrupted therapy. Enteral treatment should be resumed as soon as the patient is able to tolerate it postoperatively, and serum levels of certain drugs, such as phenytoin or valproate, should be monitored where appropriate (Klimek and Dammers 2010).

Pregnancy

Most antiepileptic drugs (AEDs) carry a degree of teratogenic risk, though the severity varies between agents. High-risk drugs include sodium valproate, phenytoin, carbamazepine and topiramate, while lower-risk alternatives such as lamotrigine and levetiracetam are generally preferred. Despite these concerns, uncontrolled seizures themselves pose significant dangers to both mother and fetus, so management should focus on maintaining seizure control while minimising fetal risk. The recommended approach is to aim for monotherapy at the lowest effective dose, and to prescribe high-dose folic acid (5 mg daily) ideally before conception and continuing throughout pregnancy (Khuda et al. 2018) (Table 6.1).

6.1.1 Levetiracetam

Levetiracetam is a broad-spectrum antiepileptic drug (AED) used in both acute and chronic seizure management. It is effective in focal seizures, generalised tonic–clonic seizures, and myoclonic seizures, and is increasingly employed for seizure prophylaxis in neurosurgical and critical care settings (Contreras García et al. 2022).

Table 6.1 Classification of anticonvulsants

Mechanism	Examples
Sodium Channel Blockers	Phenytoin, Carbamazepine, Lamotrigine
GABA Enhancement	Benzodiazepines, Phenobarbital, Valproate
Calcium Channel Blockers	Ethosuximide, Gabapentin
Synaptic Vesicle Protein Modulation	Levetiracetam
Glutamate Antagonists	Topiramate, Perampanel
Mixed/Other	Valproate (multiple mechanisms), Zonisamide

Mechanism of Action

Levetiracetam's precise mechanism remains incompletely understood, but it differs significantly from traditional AEDs. It does not block voltage-gated sodium channels or directly enhance GABAergic transmission. Instead, it binds to the synaptic vesicle protein SV2A, a membrane glycoprotein involved in neurotransmitter release. This binding modulates synaptic transmission, thereby reducing neuronal excitability and seizure propagation (Contreras García et al. 2022).

Pharmacokinetics

Levetiracetam is available in both oral and intravenous forms, with nearly complete oral bioavailability (~100%). It has minimal protein binding (<10%) and is not metabolised via the cytochrome P450 system, resulting in a low potential for drug–drug interactions. It undergoes minor enzymatic hydrolysis and is primarily excreted unchanged in the urine. The elimination half-life is approximately 7 h (Patsalos 2000).

Side Effects

Levetiracetam is generally well tolerated. Common adverse effects include fatigue, dizziness, and headache. However, neuropsychiatric symptoms are not uncommon and may include irritability, agitation, mood swings, anxiety, and rarely depression or psychosis. Suicidal ideation is a rare but recognised risk, warranting mood monitoring (Esang et al. 2020). Severe hypersensitivity reactions such as Stevens–Johnson syndrome (SJS) and toxic epidermal necrolysis (TEN) have also been reported, albeit infrequently.

Dosing

The initial recommended dose is 500 mg twice daily, administered either orally or intravenously. Maintenance therapy typically falls within the range of 500–1500 mg twice daily, with a maximum daily dose of 3000 mg. Dose titration should be undertaken gradually over 1 to 2 weeks, guided by patient tolerability and clinical response (Patsalos 2000).

Other Considerations

In patients with renal impairment, dosing requires adjustment according to creatinine clearance, whereas no modification is necessary in the presence of hepatic impairment. The drug has minimal interactions, making it particularly suitable for use in polypharmacy and critical care settings (Patsalos 2000).

6.1.2 Lamotrigine

Lamotrigine is a broad-spectrum antiepileptic drug also used in psychiatry for mood stabilisation. It is effective in the treatment of focal seizures, generalised tonic–clonic seizures, and absence seizures. Beyond epilepsy, it is licensed for maintenance therapy in bipolar disorder to prevent depressive relapses. Off-label uses include trigeminal neuralgia, migraine prophylaxis, and certain forms of neuropathic pain (Garnett 1997).

Mechanism of Action

Lamotrigine primarily acts by inhibiting voltage-gated sodium channels, thereby stabilising neuronal membranes and reducing the release of excitatory neurotransmitters such as glutamate and aspartate. This mechanism underlies both its anticonvulsant and mood-stabilising effects (Garnett 1997).

Pharmacokinetics

Administered exclusively via the oral route, lamotrigine has excellent bioavailability (~98%) and moderate protein binding (~55%). It undergoes hepatic metabolism via glucuronidation, primarily by UGT1A4 and UGT2B7, and is excreted primarily in the urine. The elimination half-life is approximately 30 h in monotherapy but may vary significantly with co-medication:

- Reduced (e.g. ~14 h) with enzyme inducers such as carbamazepine or phenytoin
- Prolonged (e.g. up to 60 h) when co-administered with valproate (Garnett 1997).

Side Effects

Rash is the most common adverse effect and may range from mild to severe. Life-threatening hypersensitivity reactions such as Stevens–Johnson Syndrome (SJS) and toxic epidermal necrolysis (TEN) are rare but more likely with rapid dose escalation or co-administration with valproate. Other adverse effects include dizziness, headache, diplopia, insomnia, and gastrointestinal upset. Leucopenia has been reported. Neuroleptic Malignant Syndrome (NMS) is rare but has occurred, particularly when combined with antipsychotic medications (Garnett 1997).

Other Considerations

Lamotrigine is considered one of the safer antiepileptics in pregnancy, with a relatively low teratogenic risk. Data from the Australian Pregnancy Register reported a malformation rate of 4.9% with lamotrigine monotherapy, which is substantially lower than the rate observed with valproate (15.2%) (Vajda et al. 2010). Dosing requires careful titration to minimise the risk of rash:

- Start low and go slow, especially if combined with valproate (which increases lamotrigine levels)
- Higher doses may be required if used with enzyme-inducing drugs such as carbamazepine, phenytoin, or phenobarbital

Typical Dosing

The initial recommended dose is 25 mg once daily, with gradual increases every 1 to 2 weeks. Maintenance therapy is usually within the range of 100–200 mg per day in divided doses, although this may vary depending on concomitant medications (Garnett 1997).

6.1.3 Phenytoin

Phenytoin is a long-established anticonvulsant with additional anti-arrhythmic properties. It is used in the treatment of focal and generalised tonic–clonic seizures, and remains a key agent in the management of status epilepticus following initial benzodiazepine therapy (Cloyd et al. 1980). It also serves as a Class Ib anti-arrhythmic, particularly effective in ventricular arrhythmias, and has been used off-label in trigeminal neuralgia refractory to first-line agents.

Mechanism of Action

Phenytoin acts by stabilising neuronal membranes through selective binding to voltage-gated sodium channels in their inactivated state. This prolongs the refractory period and inhibits repetitive high-frequency neuronal firing, thereby suppressing seizure propagation. In cardiac tissue, it shortens the action potential duration in depolarised Purkinje fibres and ventricular myocardium, forming the basis of its Class Ib anti-arrhythmic effect (Richens 1979).

Pharmacokinetics

Phenytoin is available in oral, intravenous, and rectal formulations. It has high oral bioavailability (~85%) and is extensively bound to plasma proteins (~95%), predisposing to drug–drug interactions with other highly protein-bound agents (Richens 1979). It is metabolised hepatically via CYP2C9 and CYP2C19 and exhibits zero-order (saturation) kinetics within or near the therapeutic range—meaning small dose increases can produce disproportionately large rises in serum concentration (Iorga 2023).

- Half-life: ~15 h, but highly variable due to saturable metabolism
- Excretion: Predominantly biliary, with minor renal elimination

Adverse Effects

Acute toxicity is often dose-related and includes:

- Nystagmus, ataxia, diplopia, dysarthria, and sedation
- Hypotension and arrhythmias with rapid IV administration (Cloyd et al. 1980)

Chronic use is associated with:

- Gingival hyperplasia, hirsutism, and coarsening of facial features
- Acneiform rash
- Folate deficiency with resultant macrocytic anaemia

Rare but serious adverse effects include:

- Aplastic anaemia, agranulocytosis, thrombocytopenia
- Stevens–Johnson Syndrome (SJS) and Toxic Epidermal Necrolysis (TEN), particularly in patients with HLA-B*1502 allele (common in East Asian populations)

- Drug-induced lupus erythematosus
- Teratogenicity: Associated with fetal hydantoin syndrome (craniofacial dysmorphism, neural tube defects, developmental delay) (Richens 1979; Iorga 2023)

Other Considerations

Phenytoin is a potent enzyme inducer (CYP3A4, CYP2C9), which may reduce plasma levels of numerous drugs, including warfarin, corticosteroids, and oral contraceptives (Richens 1979). Therapeutic drug monitoring is essential due to its narrow therapeutic index and non-linear pharmacokinetics.

It is contraindicated in:

- Bradycardia
- Second- or third-degree atrioventricular block
- Stokes–Adams syndrome

Also useful in certain digitalis-induced ventricular arrhythmias due to its electrophysiological effects (Cloyd et al. 1980).

Dosing

- Status epilepticus:
  - IV loading dose: 10–15 mg/kg, infused slowly over 1–4 h
  - Maximum rate: 50 mg/min to minimise risk of hypotension and arrhythmias (Cloyd et al. 1980)
- Maintenance:
  - 100 mg orally three times daily, or 300 mg once daily in well-controlled patients (Richens 1979)

6.1.4 Carbemazepine

Carbamazepine is a first-line antiepileptic agent used in the treatment of focal and generalised tonic–clonic seizures, and is the drug of choice for trigeminal neuralgia. It is also used in neuropathic pain and as a mood stabiliser in bipolar disorder, particularly for acute manic episodes. Occasionally, it is employed as an adjunct in schizoaffective disorders (Harkin 2010).

Mechanism of Action

Carbamazepine stabilises neuronal membranes by blocking voltage-gated sodium channels in their inactivated state, thereby reducing high-frequency neuronal firing. This action limits seizure propagation and also contributes to its efficacy in neuropathic pain and mood stabilisation (Harkin 2010).

Pharmacokinetics
Carbamazepine is administered orally and has excellent bioavailability (~100%). It is highly protein bound (~75%) and undergoes hepatic metabolism via CYP3A4, forming the active metabolite carbamazepine-10,11-epoxide. With continued dosing, the drug induces its own metabolism (autoinduction), shortening its half-life from approximately 36 to 20 h over a few days (Bertilsson 1978). Excretion is primarily renal, with some biliary elimination. As a strong enzyme inducer, carbamazepine accelerates the metabolism of many drugs, including warfarin, oral contraceptives, corticosteroids, and other anticonvulsants—necessitating close monitoring for interactions (Spina and Perucca 1996).

Adverse Effects
Common side effects include nausea, vomiting, dizziness, diplopia, and headache. Hyponatraemia, due to syndrome of inappropriate antidiuretic hormone secretion (SIADH), is relatively frequent, especially in elderly patients.

Serious adverse effects include:

- Haematological: aplastic anaemia, agranulocytosis, and neutropenia—routine FBC monitoring is essential.
- Dermatological: Stevens–Johnson Syndrome (SJS) and Toxic Epidermal Necrolysis (TEN), particularly in HLA-B*1502 positive individuals (screening is advised in East Asian populations).
- Hepatic: hepatotoxicity requiring periodic LFTs.
- Psychiatric: suicidal ideation, most commonly in the early phase of treatment.
- Teratogenicity: linked to spina bifida, craniofacial abnormalities, and neurodevelopmental delay (Spina and Perucca 1996).

Other Considerations
Carbamazepine is ineffective in absence seizures and is less suitable in women of childbearing age due to its teratogenic potential. Safer alternatives such as lamotrigine or levetiracetam may be preferable. Autoinduction and extensive drug–drug interactions require careful monitoring and gradual titration (Bertilsson 1978; Spina and Perucca 1996).

Dosing
Initial dose is 200 mg twice daily, titrated slowly based on clinical response. The maximum recommended dose is 1200 mg/day, divided throughout the day (Harkin 2010).

6.1.5 Sodium Valproate

Sodium valproate is a broad-spectrum antiepileptic drug used as first-line therapy for generalised seizures, including absence, myoclonic, and tonic–clonic types. It also serves as a mood stabiliser in bipolar affective disorder, and is sometimes used off-label for chronic neuropathic pain (such as trigeminal neuralgia) and migraine prophylaxis, especially in refractory cases (Zaccara et al. 1988).

Mechanism of Action
Valproate acts via several complementary mechanisms. It increases synaptic GABA concentrations by inhibiting GABA transaminase and succinic semialdehyde dehydrogenase, thereby enhancing inhibitory neurotransmission. In addition, it blocks voltage-gated sodium channels, reducing neuronal excitability, and inhibits T-type calcium channels, a mechanism particularly relevant in absence seizures. This multifaceted mode of action explains its effectiveness across various seizure types (Zaccara et al. 1988).

Pharmacokinetics
Sodium valproate is well absorbed orally, with nearly 100% bioavailability. It is highly protein-bound (~90%) and undergoes extensive hepatic metabolism, primarily through glucuronidation and mitochondrial β-oxidation. The elimination half-life is around 12 h but can be prolonged in overdose or liver dysfunction. It is excreted mainly via the urine, with some biliary elimination. At high doses, protein binding sites become saturated, resulting in non-linear kinetics (Zaccara et al. 1988).

Adverse Effects
Common side effects include gastrointestinal upset (nausea, vomiting, abdominal pain), sedation, dizziness, tremor, weight gain, and hair thinning or curling.

Serious complications include:

- Hepatotoxicity, which carries a black-box warning. Risk is highest in children under 2 years and those on polytherapy. Baseline and periodic liver function tests are essential.
- Acute pancreatitis, although rare, may be life-threatening.
- Hyperammonaemic encephalopathy, particularly when used with topiramate.
- Thrombocytopenia and coagulopathies.
- Teratogenicity is significant, with increased risks of spina bifida, craniofacial anomalies, and neurodevelopmental delay (Jentink et al. 2010; Koren et al. 2006).

Other Considerations
Due to its teratogenic profile, valproate use is contraindicated in pregnancy unless no effective alternative exists. In women of childbearing potential, it should only be prescribed with appropriate risk acknowledgement, informed consent, and regular pregnancy testing (Jentink et al. 2010). Routine therapeutic drug monitoring is typically unnecessary but may be considered in suspected toxicity or

non-compliance. Valproate also inhibits CYP2C9, potentially increasing serum levels of lamotrigine, phenobarbital, and other drugs. Protein-binding interactions may occur with warfarin, phenytoin, and aspirin (Zaccara et al. 1988).

Dosing
Initial dosing typically starts at 300–600 mg/day in divided doses, titrated according to clinical response. Maintenance doses range from 1000 to 2000 mg/day, with maximum daily doses of up to 2500 mg in selected cases (Zaccara et al. 1988).

6.2 Antidepressant Drugs

Antidepressants are a diverse group of medications primarily indicated for the treatment of major depressive disorder, anxiety disorders, and increasingly, chronic pain syndromes. Their pharmacological actions are centred on modulating monoamine neurotransmitters—serotonin (5-HT), noradrenaline (NA), and dopamine (DA)—which play key roles in regulating mood, arousal, and affect.

The Monoamine Hypothesis remains a foundational concept in psychopharmacology, proposing that depression is associated with deficient levels of serotonin, noradrenaline, and dopamine within synaptic clefts (Schildkraut 1965). Antidepressants exert their therapeutic effects by inhibiting reuptake (e.g. SSRIs, SNRIs, TCAs), blocking enzymatic breakdown (e.g. MAOIs), or modulating pre- and post-synaptic receptors to enhance neurotransmitter availability and signalling. While generally safe and effective, antidepressants are associated with a characteristic side effect profile. Common adverse effects across classes include sexual dysfunction, gastrointestinal upset (nausea, diarrhoea), weight changes, insomnia or sedation, and hyponatraemia (particularly in the elderly). Cardiac effects, such as QT interval prolongation, are most notable with citalopram and tricyclic antidepressants (TCAs).

Serotonin Syndrome
A rare but potentially fatal complication caused by excess serotonergic activity, particularly in patients receiving multiple serotonergic agents (e.g. SSRIs combined with MAOIs, SNRIs, or certain opioids such as tramadol or fentanyl). Clinical features include:

- Altered mental status (confusion, agitation)
- Autonomic instability (e.g. hyperthermia, tachycardia)
- Neuromuscular excitation (clonus, hyperreflexia) (Boyer and Shannon 2005).

Discontinuation Syndrome
Abrupt cessation of SSRIs, SNRIs, or TCAs can lead to a transient but distressing withdrawal state. Symptoms include:

- Flu-like malaise
- Sensory disturbances (commonly described as "brain zaps")
- Anxiety, irritability, and insomnia

Prevention involves gradual dose tapering over several weeks, particularly for agents with short half-lives (e.g. paroxetine, venlafaxine) (Warner et al. 2006) (Table 6.2).

Table 6.2 Classes of antidepressants

Class	Examples	Mechanism of action	Clinical notes
Selective Serotonin Reuptake Inhibitors (SSRIs)	Fluoxetine, Sertraline, Citalopram	Inhibit serotonin reuptake at the synapse	First-line for depression and anxiety; fewer side effects than older drugs
Serotonin-Norepinephrine Reuptake Inhibitors (SNRIs)	Venlafaxine, Duloxetine	Inhibit both serotonin and noradrenaline reuptake	Useful in neuropathic pain; monitor for increased BP
Norepinephrine Reuptake Inhibitors (NERIs)	Reboxetine	Selectively inhibit NA reuptake	Less commonly used; may cause insomnia and anxiety
Norepinephrine-Dopamine Reuptake Inhibitors (NDRIs)	Bupropion	Inhibits NA and DA reuptake	Less sexual dysfunction; useful in smoking cessation; avoid in epilepsy
Tricyclic Antidepressants (TCAs)	Amitriptyline, Nortriptyline	Inhibit reuptake of 5-HT and NA; also block H1, M1, α1 receptors	Effective but many side effects (sedation, arrhythmia, weight gain)
Tetracyclic Antidepressants (TeCAs)	Mirtazapine	α2-antagonist; enhances release of 5-HT and NA	Sedating at low doses; less sexual dysfunction
Monoamine Oxidase Inhibitors (MAOIs)	Phenelzine, Tranylcypromine	Inhibit monoamine oxidase enzymes (A & B) that degrade 5-HT, NA, DA	Dietary restrictions (tyramine); many interactions; rarely first-line
NMDA Receptor Antagonists	Esketamine (intranasal)	Modulates glutamatergic system via NMDA antagonism	Used in treatment-resistant depression; rapid onset of action

6.2.1 Selective Serotonin Reuptake Inhibitors (SSRIs)

Examples: Sertraline, Fluoxetine, Citalopram, Paroxetine, Escitalopram

Clinical Uses
SSRIs are widely considered first-line pharmacological therapy for a broad range of psychiatric and functional disorders. Their favourable safety profile, efficacy, and tolerability make them the mainstay for conditions including:

- Major depressive disorder
- Generalised anxiety disorder
- Post-traumatic stress disorder (PTSD)
- Obsessive-compulsive disorder (OCD)
- Panic disorder and social anxiety disorder
- Bulimia nervosa and binge-eating disorders
- Premenstrual dysphoric disorder
- Chronic pain syndromes (adjunctive role) (Preskorn 1997).

Mechanism of Action
SSRIs selectively block the serotonin transporter (SERT) on presynaptic neurons, inhibiting the reuptake of serotonin (5-HT) from the synaptic cleft. This results in increased synaptic serotonin concentration and enhanced serotonergic neurotransmission. Their relative selectivity for serotonin over noradrenaline and dopamine pathways underlies their favourable tolerability when compared with older antidepressants (Preskorn 1997).

Pharmacokinetics
Pharmacokinetic properties vary by drug. For example, escitalopram is orally administered with ~80% bioavailability and ~50–80% protein binding. SSRIs are primarily metabolised in the liver via CYP3A4, CYP2C19, and CYP2D6 pathways. Half-lives differ significantly: fluoxetine has an elimination half-life of 4–6 days (plus active metabolite), while others such as sertraline and citalopram range from 20 to 35 h. Most agents reach steady-state within 1 week (van Harten 1993).

Adverse Effects
While generally well tolerated, selective serotonin reuptake inhibitors (SSRIs) are associated with a range of common and dose-related adverse effects. Gastrointestinal disturbances such as nausea, diarrhoea and appetite changes are frequently reported, while sexual dysfunction—including reduced libido, anorgasmia and erectile dysfunction—is highly prevalent though often underreported (Fava and Rankin 2002). Neuropsychiatric effects may also occur, particularly during initiation, including agitation, insomnia, akathisia and paradoxical anxiety, with an increased risk of suicidal thoughts in adolescents and young adults. Hyponatraemia secondary to SIADH is an important concern in older adults. Other recognised effects include

sleep disturbances such as vivid dreams or insomnia, weight gain with prolonged use, photosensitivity and mild dermatological reactions. Rare but serious complications include serotonin syndrome, especially when combined with other serotonergic agents, and discontinuation syndrome characterised by dizziness, anxiety, "brain zaps" and flu-like symptoms, most commonly seen with paroxetine or sertraline (Preskorn 1997; van Harten 1993).

Clinical Considerations

SSRIs are safe in overdose and preferred in populations at risk of self-harm. However, caution is warranted in patients taking anticoagulants, NSAIDs, or antiplatelet agents, as SSRIs may impair platelet aggregation and increase bleeding risk. They should be tapered slowly when discontinuing therapy to avoid withdrawal symptoms. Importantly, SSRIs may take 2–4 weeks to exert full therapeutic effect. Adherence counselling is essential during this initiation phase to mitigate early drop-out due to transient side effects (Preskorn 1997) (Table 6.3).

6.2.2 Serotonin-Norepinephrine Reuptake Inhibitors (SNRIs)

Examples: Duloxetine, Venlafaxine, Desvenlafaxine, Milnacipran, Levomilnacipran

Clinical Uses

SNRIs are second-generation antidepressants used to treat a wide spectrum of psychiatric and chronic pain disorders. They are licensed for:

- Major depressive disorder (MDD)
- Generalised anxiety disorder (GAD)
- Obsessive-compulsive disorder (OCD)
- Attention-deficit hyperactivity disorder (ADHD)
- Chronic pain conditions including diabetic neuropathy, fibromyalgia, and musculoskeletal pain (e.g. osteoarthritis, chronic back pain)

Their efficacy in both mood regulation and analgesia makes them particularly valuable in patients with comorbid depression and chronic pain (Ormseth et al. 2011).

Table 6.3 SSRI dosage examples

Drug	Starting dose	Maximum dose
Sertraline	50 mg once daily	200 mg/day
Escitalopram	10 mg once daily	20 mg/day
Fluoxetine	20 mg once daily	80 mg/day
Citalopram	20 mg once daily	40 mg/day
Paroxetine	20 mg once daily	50 mg/day

Mechanism of Action

SNRIs inhibit the presynaptic reuptake of serotonin (5-HT) and noradrenaline (NA), increasing their concentration in the synaptic cleft. This dual action enhances mood and augments descending inhibitory pain pathways. At higher doses, venlafaxine and desvenlafaxine may also weakly inhibit dopamine reuptake, although the clinical significance of this is limited (de Vries and Schoemaker 2004).

Pharmacokinetics

SNRIs are administered orally and undergo extensive hepatic metabolism, primarily via CYP2D6 and CYP1A2 (notably for duloxetine). Their active metabolites contribute to prolonged clinical effects. Venlafaxine has a relatively short half-life (~5 h), but its metabolite O-desmethylvenlafaxine extends the overall pharmacological activity (~11 h). Duloxetine has a half-life of approximately 12 h. Steady-state plasma levels are generally reached within 2–3 days of consistent dosing (de Vries and Schoemaker 2004).

Adverse Effects

Side effects are often dose-dependent and more prominent during the initiation phase. Gastrointestinal symptoms such as nausea, vomiting, and reduced appetite are common. Headache, dizziness, insomnia, and anxiety may also occur. Sexual dysfunction (e.g. anorgasmia, erectile dysfunction) is a frequent reason for treatment discontinuation. SNRIs may cause hypertension, particularly at higher doses of venlafaxine, and are associated with increased bleeding risk when combined with NSAIDs or anticoagulants. As with all antidepressants, a temporary increase in suicidal ideation may occur in younger patients at the start of therapy. Serotonin syndrome is a rare but serious complication, especially in the context of polypharmacy with other serotonergic agents (Shelton 2009).

Clinical Considerations

SNRIs should be avoided in patients with recent monoamine oxidase inhibitor (MAOI) use due to the risk of serotonin syndrome. Caution is advised in those with coronary artery disease or uncontrolled hypertension. Discontinuation syndrome is well recognised, particularly with venlafaxine, and can include dizziness, insomnia, irritability, and sensory disturbances ("brain zaps"). To minimise this, SNRIs should be tapered gradually rather than stopped abruptly (Shelton 2009) (Table 6.4).

Table 6.4 SNRI dosing

Drug	Starting dose	Maximum dose
Duloxetine	20–30 mg twice daily	120 mg/day (usually split dose)
Venlafaxine	37.5 mg once or twice daily	225–250 mg/day (in divided doses)
(Extended-release forms allow for once-daily dosing)		

6.2.3 Monoamine Oxidase Inhibitors (MAOIs)

Examples

- Non-selective (MAO-A & B): Phenelzine, Tranylcypromine
- MAO-A selective: Moclobemide
- MAO-B selective: Selegiline, Rasagiline

Clinical Uses

MAOIs are typically reserved for treatment-resistant or atypical depression, especially when other classes of antidepressants have failed (Thase 1995). They are occasionally used for panic disorder, PTSD, and bipolar depression. MAO-B selective inhibitors such as selegiline and rasagiline are more commonly employed in Parkinson's disease to enhance central dopaminergic tone (Finberg and Gillman 2011).

Mechanism of Action

Monoamine oxidase (MAO) is an intracellular enzyme responsible for the breakdown of monoamine neurotransmitters such as serotonin, noradrenaline, and dopamine. MAO-A preferentially metabolises serotonin and noradrenaline, while MAO-B predominantly metabolises dopamine. MAOIs increase synaptic concentrations of these neurotransmitters by inhibiting this enzymatic degradation:

- MAO-A inhibition → increases serotonin, noradrenaline, and dopamine
- MAO-B inhibition → increases dopamine (predominantly)

Irreversible inhibitors (e.g. phenelzine) bind covalently and require enzyme regeneration after discontinuation, whereas moclobemide, a reversible MAO-A inhibitor, has a shorter duration and improved safety profile (Yamada and Yasuhara 2004).

Pharmacokinetics

MAOIs are primarily administered orally, though selegiline is also available as a transdermal patch and sublingual tablet. Oral bioavailability is variable due to extensive first-pass metabolism. These drugs are metabolised hepatically (via acetylation and oxidation), and their half-lives differ significantly between agents: moclobemide has a half-life of ~2 h, while phenelzine has a longer half-life of ~11 h. Despite this, irreversible inhibitors have prolonged pharmacodynamic effects, with enzyme inhibition persisting for 7–14 days after cessation (Yamada and Yasuhara 2004).

Adverse Effects

MAOIs are associated with a range of systemic and potentially serious side effects:

- Hypertensive crisis following ingestion of tyramine-rich foods (e.g. aged cheese, cured meats)—the so-called cheese reaction (Finberg and Gillman 2011)

- Serotonin syndrome when used with other serotonergic agents
- Orthostatic hypotension, especially in elderly patients
- Insomnia, agitation, tremor, and dry mouth
- Weight gain, particularly with phenelzine
- Sexual dysfunction
- Withdrawal symptoms on abrupt discontinuation
- Exaggerated hypertensive response to vasopressors such as adrenaline or ephedrine

Clinical Considerations

Non-selective and irreversible MAOIs necessitate strict dietary restrictions to avoid tyramine-induced hypertensive crisis (Finberg and Gillman 2011). Drug–drug interactions are numerous and potentially life-threatening, particularly with SSRIs, SNRIs, TCAs, opioids (notably pethidine and tramadol), and sympathomimetics. A minimum 14-day washout is recommended when switching from irreversible MAOIs to other serotonergic or noradrenergic antidepressants (Yamada and Yasuhara 2004). Moclobemide, a reversible MAO-A inhibitor, poses fewer risks and does not require dietary restrictions, making it a safer option in some cases (Table 6.5).

6.2.4 Tricyclic Antidepressants (TCAs)

Examples: Amitriptyline, Nortriptyline, Imipramine, Clomipramine, Desipramine, Doxepin

Clinical Uses

Tricyclic antidepressants (TCAs) are an older class of antidepressants now less commonly used for depression due to their adverse effect profile and overdose toxicity. However, they remain clinically valuable for a variety of psychiatric and somatic conditions. These include major depressive disorder, anxiety disorders (such as panic disorder and generalised anxiety disorder), obsessive-compulsive disorder (particularly clomipramine), and post-traumatic stress disorder. They are also effective in managing chronic neuropathic pain, fibromyalgia, migraine

Table 6.5 MAO-I dosage examples

Drug	Dose range	Notes
Moclobemide	300–600 mg/day (divided doses)	Reversible, selective MAO-A inhibitor; safer interaction profile
Phenelzine	15–90 mg/day (divided doses)	Non-selective, irreversible MAOI—high risk of dietary interactions
Selegiline	5–10 mg/day (oral) or 6–12 mg/24 h (patch)	Selective MAO-B inhibitor—often used in Parkinson's disease

prophylaxis, and nocturnal enuresis (especially with imipramine in children) (Sindrup and Jensen 1999). Off-label uses extend to eating disorders, ADHD, and some personality disorders (Schneider 2019).

Mechanism of Action
TCAs act primarily by inhibiting the presynaptic reuptake of noradrenaline and serotonin through blockade of their respective transporters (NET and SERT), increasing synaptic concentrations and enhancing mood regulation. In addition to this core mechanism, TCAs antagonise multiple receptor types—including muscarinic (M1), histamine (H1), and alpha-1 adrenergic receptors—which contributes to both therapeutic and adverse effects. Some TCAs also modulate glutamate via NMDA receptor antagonism and may act as sigma receptor agonists (Gillman 2007).

Pharmacokinetics
All TCAs are administered orally (some also intramuscularly) and are highly protein-bound (~95%). Their oral bioavailability is moderate (~50%) due to extensive first-pass hepatic metabolism. Amitriptyline, for example, is metabolised by CYP2D6 to its active form nortriptyline. The half-life is variable (typically 15–40 h), and excretion is primarily renal. CYP2D6 polymorphisms can influence plasma drug levels and side effect burden (Gillman 2007).

Adverse Effects
The diverse receptor profile of TCAs underlies a wide range of side effects. Anticholinergic effects—such as dry mouth, blurred vision, constipation, urinary retention, and cognitive impairment—are common. H1 antagonism leads to sedation and weight gain, while alpha-1 blockade can cause orthostatic hypotension and dizziness. Cardiac toxicity is a serious concern: sodium channel blockade may result in tachycardia, QT prolongation, and ventricular arrhythmias, particularly in overdose. Other neurological effects include seizures and tremor, and sexual dysfunction is also common. Abrupt cessation may cause withdrawal symptoms (discontinuation syndrome), and overdose can be fatal, especially in combination with alcohol or other CNS depressants (Gillman 2007).

Clinical Considerations
Due to their high lethality in overdose, TCAs require careful prescribing—particularly in patients at risk of self-harm. They are often dosed at night due to their sedating properties. TCAs interact with many other drugs through CYP2D6 and should be used cautiously alongside SSRIs, MAOIs, and other QT-prolonging agents. They are generally avoided in patients with significant cardiovascular disease (Schneider 2019). CYP2D6 polymorphisms may necessitate dose adjustments or therapeutic drug monitoring (Gillman 2007).

Table 6.6 TCA dosage examples

Drug	Starting dose	Max dose	Notes
Amitriptyline	75 mg/day (divided or nocte)	300 mg/day	Often used at lower doses for chronic pain
Imipramine	75 mg once daily	200 mg/day	Used in depression and nocturnal enuresis
Doxepin	75 mg/day (divided or once daily)	150 mg/day	Can be used at very low doses (3–6 mg) for insomnia

Dosing (e.g. Amitriptyline)
Initial dosing typically starts at 25–50 mg at night, with gradual titration to 75–150 mg/day. For neuropathic pain or migraine, lower doses (10–25 mg at night) are often sufficient. Elderly or frail patients may require more conservative initiation and slower titration (Sindrup and Jensen 1999) (Table 6.6).

6.2.5 Tetracyclic Antidepressants (TeCAs)

Examples: Mirtazapine, Maprotiline

Clinical Uses
TeCAs are most commonly prescribed for major depressive disorder, particularly when associated with insomnia, poor appetite, or anxiety. Mirtazapine is also used in generalised anxiety disorder, post-traumatic stress disorder (off-label), and social anxiety disorder. Its appetite-stimulating and sedative properties make it especially useful in palliative care or for patients with cancer-related cachexia or significant weight loss (Davis and Wilde 1996).

Mechanism of Action
Unlike SSRIs and TCAs, mirtazapine does not inhibit serotonin reuptake. Instead, it acts as an antagonist at central presynaptic α_2-adrenergic autoreceptors and heteroreceptors, leading to enhanced noradrenaline and serotonin release. It also blocks 5-HT_2 and 5-HT_3 receptors, thereby enhancing 5-HT_1-mediated neurotransmission, which contributes to its antidepressant and anxiolytic effects while minimising gastrointestinal and sexual side effects (Anttila and Leinonen 2001). Its potent antagonism of histamine H_1 receptors underlies its sedative profile (Davis and Wilde 1996).

Pharmacokinetics (Mirtazapine)
Mirtazapine is administered orally with a bioavailability of approximately 50%. It is highly protein-bound (~85%) and undergoes hepatic metabolism via CYP1A2, CYP2D6, and CYP3A4 pathways. The elimination half-life ranges from 20 to 40 h, allowing once-daily dosing, and the drug is excreted via both urine and faeces (Timmer 2000).

Table 6.7 TeCA dosage examples

Drug	Starting dose	Maximum dose
Mirtazapine	15 mg once daily (at night)	45 mg/day
Maprotiline	75 mg/day	150–225 mg/day (in divided doses)

Adverse Effects

Sedation and weight gain are the most notable side effects, often regarded as therapeutic in underweight or agitated patients. Appetite stimulation occurs via H_1 and 5-HT_2C antagonism (Anttila and Leinonen 2001). Other side effects include dry mouth, dizziness, constipation, and—rarely—agranulocytosis. Unlike SSRIs and SNRIs, mirtazapine causes minimal sexual dysfunction and carries a lower risk of serotonin syndrome, making it a favourable option for many patients (Davis and Wilde 1996).

Clinical Considerations

Mirtazapine is well-suited for patients experiencing SSRI-induced insomnia, anorexia, or sexual dysfunction. It has a lower toxicity profile in overdose compared to TCAs. For treatment-resistant depression, it can be used in combination with SSRIs or SNRIs as part of augmentation strategies (Anttila and Leinonen 2001). Abrupt cessation should be avoided to prevent rebound anxiety or insomnia; tapering is advised (Timmer 2000) (Table 6.7).

6.3 Hypnotic Drugs

6.3.1 Benzodiazepines

Benzodiazepines are psychoactive compounds widely used across clinical specialties for their sedative, anxiolytic, muscle relaxant, hypnotic, and anticonvulsant properties. First introduced with the synthesis of chlordiazepoxide in 1955, they have since become among the most commonly prescribed CNS depressants. Their clinical versatility spans anaesthesia, psychiatry, neurology, emergency medicine, and intensive care (Wick 2013).

Clinical Uses

Benzodiazepines are indicated in a variety of acute and chronic settings:

- Acute seizure management, including status epilepticus
- Alcohol withdrawal, especially in preventing delirium tremens
- Generalised anxiety disorder and panic attacks
- Short-term management of insomnia
- Pre-operative anxiolysis and procedural sedation

- Muscle spasticity in conditions like multiple sclerosis
- Sedation in critical care, particularly for ventilated patients (Edwards and Preuss 2024)

Mechanism of Action

Benzodiazepines act as positive allosteric modulators at the GABA-A receptor, a ligand-gated chloride channel in the CNS. By increasing the frequency of chloride channel opening in the presence of GABA, they promote membrane hyperpolarisation and reduce neuronal excitability. This potentiation of inhibitory GABAergic signalling underlies their broad pharmacological effects. Unlike barbiturates, benzodiazepines do not activate the GABA-A receptor directly (Edwards and Preuss 2024).

Pharmacokinetics

These agents are highly lipophilic, facilitating rapid CNS penetration. Route of administration varies by agent and includes oral, intravenous, buccal, rectal, and intranasal.

Metabolism is primarily hepatic:

- CYP450 metabolism (e.g. diazepam) can lead to active metabolites and drug interactions.
- Lorazepam, temazepam, and oxazepam undergo glucuronidation and are preferred in hepatic impairment.
- Half-lives vary significantly. Diazepam and chlordiazepoxide form long-acting metabolites, while midazolam is ultra-short-acting (Griffin et al. 2013) (Table 6.8).

Adverse Effects

Benzodiazepines are generally well tolerated in the short term, but adverse effects are common, especially with prolonged use. CNS effects include sedation, drowsiness, ataxia, cognitive impairment, and anterograde amnesia (Edinoff et al. 2021). Respiratory depression may occur, particularly in combination with opioids or in vulnerable patients such as those with obstructive sleep apnoea or the elderly (Edinoff et al. 2021). Paradoxical reactions—such as agitation, aggression, and disinhibition—can arise, especially in children or older adults (Mancuso et al. 2004).

Table 6.8 Pharmacokinetics of Benzodiazepines

Classification	Example	Half-life
Short-acting (1–12 h)	Midazolam	1.5–2.5 h
Intermediate (12–40 h)	Lorazepam, Alprazolam, Temazepam	10–20 h
Long-acting (40+ h)	Diazepam, Chlordiazepoxide, Clonazepam, Oxazepam	40–80 h+

Long-term complications include tolerance, dependence, withdrawal, rebound anxiety or insomnia, and chronic cognitive slowing (Ashton 2005). Sexual dysfunction and hypotension may also occur (Edinoff et al. 2021).

Clinical Considerations

Withdrawal may begin after just 2–4 weeks of regular use and can be severe. Symptoms include tremor, anxiety, insomnia, hallucinations, and seizures (Ashton 2005). Gradual tapering is essential, with long-acting agents such as diazepam or chlordiazepoxide typically used in detoxification protocols (Ashton 2005). Overdose usually results from co-ingestion with alcohol or opioids and manifests as CNS depression, hypotension, and respiratory compromise (Edinoff et al. 2021). Flumazenil, a competitive GABA-A antagonist, can reverse benzodiazepine effects but must be used cautiously due to the risk of precipitating seizures, especially in chronic users or mixed overdoses (Edinoff et al. 2021). In status epilepticus, first-line therapy includes lorazepam (0.1 mg/kg IV) or midazolam (10 mg buccal/intranasal) if IV access is unavailable. For alcohol withdrawal, long-acting agents like chlordiazepoxide reduce seizure risk and symptom severity (Ashton 2005).

Regulatory and Abuse Potential

Benzodiazepines are classified as Schedule IV controlled substances due to their potential for misuse, dependence, and recreational abuse. Euphoria and disinhibition contribute to their popularity in non-medical settings, warranting close prescribing supervision (Edinoff et al. 2021) (Table 6.9).

6.3.2 Z-Drugs

Z-drugs are non-benzodiazepine hypnotics used primarily for the short-term treatment of insomnia. Despite being chemically distinct from benzodiazepines, they share a similar mechanism of action at the GABA-A receptor, producing sedative and hypnotic effects. Common agents include zolpidem, zopiclone, and zaleplon. They are favoured for their rapid onset and short duration of action, allowing effective sleep induction with minimal residual sedation. However, concerns persist

Table 6.9 Benzodiazepine equivalency chart

Drug	Approximate equivalent to diazepam 10 mg	Half-life (hours)	Comments
Midazolam	5 mg	1.5–2.5	Rapid onset, short duration
Lorazepam	1–2 mg	10–20	Preferred in seizures
Temazepam	20 mg	8–15	Hypnotic
Diazepam	10 mg	20–80	Long-acting with active metabolites
Chlordiazepoxide	25 mg	50–100	Long-acting, good for alcohol withdrawal
Clonazepam	0.5–1 mg	30–40	Potent, often used in epilepsy

regarding tolerance, dependence, cognitive side effects, and complex behaviours such as sleepwalking or sleep-driving (Gunja 2013).

Mechanism of Action

Z-drugs are positive allosteric modulators at the GABA-A receptor, binding selectively to the α1 subunit, which is associated primarily with sedation. Unlike benzodiazepines, they have minimal activity at subunits responsible for anxiolytic, muscle-relaxant, or anticonvulsant effects. This selective action accounts for their primary use in sleep disorders, but not for anxiety or epilepsy (Richter et al. 2020).

Pharmacokinetics

Z-drugs are administered orally and are rapidly absorbed, with onset of action typically within 30 min. They are hepatically metabolised, mainly via CYP3A4, and eliminated through renal excretion as inactive metabolites. Their half-lives vary:

- Zolpidem: ~2–3 h
- Zopiclone: ~5–6 h
- Zaleplon: ~1 h

This short half-life reduces next-day sedation but increases the risk of rebound insomnia upon discontinuation (Terzano et al. 2003).

Adverse Effects

The most common side effects include daytime drowsiness, headache, dry mouth, nausea, and impaired coordination. Anterograde amnesia is well documented, particularly with higher doses. Other notable risks include parasomnias, such as sleepwalking and sleep-driving, mood changes including depression and suicidal ideation, falls and fractures in older adults due to impaired balance, and cognitive impairment with chronic use (Gunja 2013).

Dependence, Withdrawal & Overdose

Dependence may occur after just 2–4 weeks of regular use. Withdrawal symptoms include rebound insomnia, anxiety, agitation, and in rare cases, seizures. Tapering is advised when discontinuing long-term therapy (Terzano et al. 2003). Overdose typically presents with profound sedation, respiratory depression, hypotension, and potentially coma—especially when combined with alcohol or opioids Flumazenil may reverse Z-drug effects but should be used with caution, particularly in mixed overdoses or patients with chronic use, due to the risk of precipitating seizures (Gunja 2013) (Table 6.10).

Table 6.10 Z-drug dosage examples

Drug	Starting dose	Maximum dose	Timing
Zolpidem	5 mg orally NOCTE	10 mg/day	Immediately before sleep
Zopiclone	3.75 mg orally NOCTE	15 mg/day	Immediately before sleep

Conflicts of Interest The authors have no conflicts of interest to declare that are relevant to the content of this chapter.

References

Anttila, S.A. and Leinonen, E.V. (2001) 'A review of the pharmacological and clinical profile of mirtazapine', *CNS Drug Reviews*, 7(3), pp. 249–264. https://doi.org/10.1111/j.1527-3458.2001.tb00198.x.

Ashton, H. (2005) 'The diagnosis and management of benzodiazepine dependence', *Current Opinion in Psychiatry*, 18(3), pp. 249–255. https://doi.org/10.1097/01.yco.0000165594.60434.84.

Bertilsson, L. (1978) 'Clinical pharmacokinetics of carbamazepine', *British Journal of Clinical Pharmacology*, 5(Suppl 4), pp. 215S–220S.

Boyer, E.W. and Shannon, M. (2005) 'The serotonin syndrome', *New England Journal of Medicine*, 352(11), pp. 1112–1120.

Cloyd, J.C., Gumnit, R.J. and Lesar, T.S. (1980). Reduced seizure control due to spoiled phenytoin capsules. *Annals of Neurology*, 7(2), pp. 191–193. https://doi.org/10.1002/ana.410070218.

Contreras García, I.J., et al. (2022) 'Levetiracetam mechanisms of action: from molecules to systems', *Pharmaceuticals*, 15(5), 550.

Davis, R. and Wilde, M.I. (1996) 'Mirtazapine: a review of its pharmacology and therapeutic potential in the management of major depression', *CNS Drugs*, 5(5), pp. 389–402.

de Vries, E.F.J. and Schoemaker, R.C. (2004) 'Clinical pharmacokinetics of venlafaxine', *Clinical Pharmacokinetics*, 43(7), pp. 443–460.

Edinoff, A.N., Nix, C.A., Hollier, J., Nix, T., Murnane, K.S., Trosclair, K., Cornett, E.M., Kaye, A.M. and Kaye, A.D. (2021) 'Benzodiazepines: uses, dangers, and clinical considerations', *Pharmaceuticals*, 14(7), 589. https://doi.org/10.3390/ph14070589.

Edwards, Z. and Preuss, C.V. (2024) 'GABA receptor positive allosteric modulators', in *StatPearls* [Internet]. Treasure Island (FL): StatPearls Publishing. Available at: https://www.ncbi.nlm.nih.gov/books/NBK554443/ (Accessed: 1 September 2025).

Esang, M.D., Santos, M.G. and Ahmed, S. (2020) 'Levetiracetam and suicidality: a case report and literature review', *Primary Care Companion for CNS Disorders*, 22(4), 19nr02502.

Fava, M. and Rankin, M. (2002) 'Sexual functioning and SSRIs', *Journal of Clinical Psychiatry*, 63(Suppl 5), pp. 13–16.

Finberg, J.P. and Gillman, K. (2011) 'Selective inhibitors of monoamine oxidase type B and the "cheese effect"', *International Review of Neurobiology*, 100, pp. 169–190.

Garnett, W.R. (1997) "Lamotrigine: pharmacokinetics', *Journal of Child Neurology*, **12**(Suppl 1), pp. S10–S15.

Gillman, P.K. (2007) 'Tricyclic antidepressant pharmacology and therapeutic drug interactions updated', *British Journal of Pharmacology*, 151(6), pp. 737–748.

Griffin, C.E., Kaye, A.M., Bueno, F.R. and Kaye, A.D. (2013) 'Benzodiazepine pharmacology and central nervous system–mediated effects', *Ochsner Journal*, 13(2), pp. 214–223.

Gunja, N. (2013) 'The clinical and forensic toxicology of Z-drugs', *Journal of Medical Toxicology*, 9(2), pp. 155–162. https://doi.org/10.1007/s13181-013-0292-0.

Harkin, G. (2010) 'Carbamazepine: mechanisms and clinical applications', *Practical Diabetes International*, 27(5), pp. 185–188.

Iorga, A. (2023) 'Phenytoin toxicity', in *StatPearls* [Internet]. Treasure Island (FL): StatPearls Publishing.

Jentink, J., Loane, M.A., Dolk, H., et al. (2010) 'Valproic acid monotherapy in pregnancy and major congenital malformations', *New England Journal of Medicine*, 362(23), pp. 2185–2193.

Khuda, I., Khan, S. and Chand, P. (2018) 'Management of epilepsy in pregnancy: a comprehensive review', *Journal of Clinical and Diagnostic Research*, 12(1), pp. OE01–OE05.

Klimek, M. and Dammers, R. (2010) 'Antiepileptic drug therapy in the perioperative course of neurosurgical patients', *Current Opinion in Anaesthesiology*, 23(5), pp. 564–567.

Koren, G., Pastuszak, A. and Ito, S. (2006) 'Major malformations with valproic acid', *Canadian Family Physician*, 352(1), pp. 17–23.

Mancuso, C.E., Tanzi, M.G. and Gabay, M. (2004) 'Paradoxical reactions to benzodiazepines: literature review and treatment options', *Pharmacotherapy*, 24(9), pp. 1177–1185.

Ormseth, M.J., Scholz, B.A. and Boomershine, C.S. (2011) 'Duloxetine in the management of diabetic peripheral neuropathic pain', *Patient Preference and Adherence*, 5, pp. 343–356.

Patsalos, P.N. (2000) 'Pharmacokinetic profile of levetiracetam: toward ideal characteristics', *Epilepsy Research*, 44(1), pp. 1–10.

Preskorn, S.H. (1997) 'Clinically relevant pharmacology of selective serotonin reuptake inhibitors', *Clinical Pharmacokinetics*, 32(Suppl 1), pp. 1–21.

Richens, A. (1979) 'Clinical pharmacokinetics of phenytoin', *British Journal of Clinical Pharmacology*, 4(3), pp. 153–169.

Richter, G., Liao, V.W.Y., Ahring, P.K. and Chebib, M. (2020) 'The Z-drugs zolpidem, zaleplon, and eszopiclone have varying actions on human GABAA receptors containing γ1, γ2, and γ3 subunits', *Frontiers in Neuroscience*, 14, 599812. https://doi.org/10.3389/fnins.2020.599812.

Schildkraut, J.J. (1965) 'The catecholamine hypothesis of affective disorders: a review of supporting evidence', *American Journal of Psychiatry*, 122(5), pp. 509–522.

Schneider, J. (2019) 'Tricyclic antidepressants: a review of clinical uses beyond depression', *Primary Care Companion for CNS Disorders*, 21(5), 19r02526. https://doi.org/10.4088/PCC.19r02526.

Shelton, R.C. (2009) 'The nature of the discontinuation syndrome associated with antidepressant drugs', *Journal of Clinical Psychiatry*, 67(Suppl 4), pp. 3–7.

Sindrup, S.H. and Jensen, T.S. (1999) 'Efficacy of pharmacological treatments of neuropathic pain: an update and effect related to mechanism of drug action', *Pain*, 83(3), pp. 389–400.

Spina, E. and Perucca, E. (1996) 'Clinically significant pharmacokinetic drug interactions with carbamazepine: interactions with newer antiepileptic drugs', *Clinical Pharmacokinetics*, 30(3), pp. 198–213.

Terzano, M.G., Rossi, M., Palomba, V., Smerieri, A. and Parrino, L. (2003) 'New drugs for insomnia: comparative tolerability of zopiclone, zolpidem and zaleplon', *Drug Safety*, 26(4), pp. 261–282.

Thase, M.E. (1995) 'MAO inhibitors: renaissance for treatment-resistant depression', *Neuropsychopharmacology*, 12(3), pp. 185–219.

Timmer, C.J. (2000) 'Clinical pharmacokinetics of mirtazapine', *Clinical Pharmacokinetics*, 38(6), pp. 461–474.

Vajda, F.J.E., et al. (2010) 'Fetal malformation rate with lamotrigine monotherapy versus valproate', *Seizure*, 19(7), pp. 355–361.

van Harten, J. (1993) 'Clinical pharmacokinetics of selective serotonin reuptake inhibitors', *Clinical Pharmacokinetics*, 24(3), pp. 203–220.

Warner, C.H., Bobo, W., Warner, C., Reid, S. and Rachal, J. (2006) 'Antidepressant discontinuation syndrome', *American Family Physician*, 74(3), pp. 449–456.

Wick, J.Y. (2013) 'The history of benzodiazepines', *Consultant Pharmacist*, 28(9), pp. 538–548. https://doi.org/10.4140/TCP.n.2013.538.

Wiffen, P.J., Derry, S., Bell, R.F., Rice, A.S.C., Tölle, T.R., Phillips, T. and Moore, R.A. (2013) 'Gabapentin and pregabalin for neuropathic pain and fibromyalgia—an overview of Cochrane reviews', *Cochrane Database of Systematic Reviews*, (4), CD010567.

Yamada, M. and Yasuhara, H. (2004) 'Clinical pharmacology of MAO inhibitors: safety and future', *Neurotoxicology*, 25(1–2), pp. 215–221.

Zaccara, G., Messori, A. and Moroni, F. (1988) 'Clinical pharmacokinetics of valproic acid', *Clinical Pharmacokinetics*, 15(6), pp. 367–389.

Anti-Diabetic Medication

7

7.1 Anti-Diabetic Drugs

The pharmacological management of diabetes mellitus (DM) is tailored to the type of diabetes, disease progression, and the degree of residual pancreatic β-cell function. The primary therapeutic goals are to normalise blood glucose, reduce insulin resistance, preserve β-cell function, and prevent complications. Antidiabetic agents work through several mechanisms: enhancing insulin secretion, improving insulin sensitivity, reducing hepatic glucose output, decreasing renal glucose reabsorption, delaying carbohydrate absorption, and promoting satiety or weight loss (Chaudhury et al. 2017; Cabré et al. 2025). Diabetes mellitus is a chronic metabolic disorder characterised by persistent hyperglycaemia. It results from absolute or relative insulin deficiency, insulin resistance, or both. Diagnosis is confirmed by fasting plasma glucose, HbA1c, or oral glucose tolerance testing, and treatment aims to prevent both acute and long-term complications.

Types of Diabetes

Type 1 Diabetes Mellitus (T1DM) is caused by autoimmune destruction of pancreatic β-cells, typically manifesting in childhood or adolescence. However, adult-onset presentations are increasingly recognised. It is associated with HLA-DR/DQ haplotypes and other autoimmune diseases such as Addison's or Hashimoto's thyroiditis (Redondo et al. 2023). Classic symptoms include polyuria, polydipsia, weight loss, and fatigue. Diabetic ketoacidosis (DKA) may be the first presentation. Exogenous insulin is essential for survival and is delivered as multiple daily injections or via continuous subcutaneous insulin infusion.

Type 2 Diabetes Mellitus (T2DM) accounts for the majority of diabetes cases and usually presents in adulthood. It is characterised by peripheral insulin resistance and relative β-cell dysfunction, commonly associated with obesity, metabolic syndrome, and a strong family history. T2DM may remain asymptomatic for years and is often diagnosed through routine screening. Management begins with lifestyle

G. Browne, *PharmacologyPro*, https://doi.org/10.1007/978-3-032-10227-0_7

modification (diet, exercise, weight reduction) and progresses to oral hypoglycaemic agents and insulin therapy if glycaemic control deteriorates (Chaudhury et al. 2017; Cabré et al. 2025). HbA1c targets are typically <7.0–7.5% but should be individualised (Table 7.1).

Antidiabetic Drug Classes

Treatment options have expanded beyond insulin and sulfonylureas to include multiple pharmacological classes. Biguanides (e.g. metformin) remain the first-line therapy in most patients with type 2 diabetes mellitus (T2DM) (Dutta et al. 2021). Sulfonylureas (e.g. gliclazide) act by increasing endogenous insulin secretion, while thiazolidinediones (e.g. pioglitazone) improve insulin sensitivity. DPP-4 inhibitors (e.g. sitagliptin) enhance incretin action, and GLP-1 receptor agonists (e.g. liraglutide) promote glucose-dependent insulin secretion, delay gastric emptying, and aid weight loss. SGLT2 inhibitors (e.g. empagliflozin) lower renal glucose reabsorption, promote glycosuria, and confer proven cardiovascular and renal protection (Zhang et al. 2022). Insulins remain the cornerstone for type 1 diabetes mellitus (T1DM) and advanced T2DM, available in rapid-, intermediate-, and long-acting formulations.

Insulin Therapy

All patients with T1DM require lifelong insulin therapy. In T2DM, insulin is typically introduced in cases of marked hyperglycaemia, failure of oral agents, or during acute illness. Insulin lowers glucose by promoting peripheral uptake—mainly in skeletal muscle—and inhibiting hepatic gluconeogenesis. Concomitant metformin is often continued in T2DM patients on insulin to improve insulin sensitivity and limit weight gain (Dutta et al. 2021).

Complications and Risk Reduction

The most serious long-term consequences of diabetes are macrovascular complications, including ischaemic heart disease, cerebrovascular disease, and peripheral arterial disease. These are the leading causes of morbidity and mortality in T2DM. Effective management requires multifactorial risk reduction, including

Table 7.1 Classification of glucose dysregulation

Category	Criteria
Diabetes Mellitus	Fasting plasma glucose ≥ 7.0 mmol/L OR Random glucose ≥ 11.1 mmol/L with symptoms (polyuria, polydipsia, weight loss) OR HbA1c ≥ 6.5%
Impaired Glucose Tolerance (IGT)	Fasting glucose < 7.0 mmol/L 2-h post-OGTT glucose 7.8–11.0 mmol/L
Impaired Fasting Glucose (IFG)	Fasting glucose 6.1–6.9 mmol/L 2-h post-OGTT glucose < 7.8 mmol/L

IGT and IFG represent pre-diabetic states. They are managed through lifestyle interventions (diet, weight loss, physical activity), but carry a high risk of progression to overt diabetes

Table 7.2 Microvascular complications

Complication	Clinical features
Retinopathy	Microaneurysms, cotton wool spots, neovascularisation; may require laser photocoagulation
Nephropathy	Microalbuminuria progressing to proteinuria and chronic kidney disease
Neuropathy	Distal sensory loss ("glove and stocking"), autonomic dysfunction, foot ulcers

blood pressure control, lipid optimisation, smoking cessation, and regular cardiovascular monitoring (Gaede et al. 2008) (Table 7.2).

7.2 Biguanides

Example: Metformin (the only biguanide in clinical use)

Metformin is the first-line pharmacological treatment for Type 2 Diabetes Mellitus (T2DM). It is particularly effective in patients with insulin resistance, and in those who are overweight or obese, as it is weight-neutral or may even promote modest weight loss. Beyond T2DM, metformin is also used off-label in polycystic ovary syndrome (PCOS) to improve insulin sensitivity, and in prediabetes for high-risk individuals. It is sometimes used in gestational diabetes, although this is case-dependent (Sanchez-Rangel and Inzucchi 2017).

Mechanism of Action

Metformin primarily acts by reducing hepatic gluconeogenesis, lowering fasting plasma glucose levels. It also enhances peripheral glucose uptake, especially in skeletal muscle, by increasing the translocation of GLUT4 glucose transporters. Additional effects include decreased intestinal glucose absorption and improved insulin sensitivity. Unlike insulin or sulfonylureas, metformin does not stimulate insulin secretion, so it does not cause hypoglycaemia when used as monotherapy. Its molecular effects are mediated through activation of AMP-activated protein kinase (AMPK), a key cellular energy sensor that regulates glucose and lipid metabolism (Sanchez-Rangel and Inzucchi 2017).

Pharmacokinetics

Metformin is administered orally, with a bioavailability of 50–60% (reduced by food). It is not protein-bound and undergoes no hepatic metabolism. The drug is excreted unchanged by the kidneys via tubular secretion, with a half-life of 5–9 h. Steady-state concentrations are typically achieved within 24–48 h. In renal impairment, accumulation may occur, increasing the risk of toxicity (Graham et al. 2011).

Adverse Effects

The most common side effects are gastrointestinal, affecting up to 30% of patients. These include nausea, diarrhoea, flatulence, and abdominal cramps, particularly early in treatment. Slow dose titration or switching to extended-release formulations can help mitigate these symptoms. A rare but serious complication is lactic acidosis, with a high mortality rate. This risk is increased in the setting of renal impairment, hepatic dysfunction, sepsis, alcohol misuse, or hypoperfusion states such as shock (Tahrani et al. 2007). Metformin has also been associated with vitamin B12 deficiency in long-term use due to impaired absorption (Graham et al. 2011).

Clinical Considerations
Metformin is contraindicated in patients with:

- eGFR <30 mL/min/1.73 m^2
- Unstable heart failure, acute illness, or hypoxia
- Chronic alcohol abuse

It should also be temporarily withheld around procedures involving IV contrast if renal function is at risk of acute decline. Metformin is not suitable for patients with Type 1 Diabetes or advanced T2DM with minimal residual β-cell function (Tahrani et al. 2007).

Dosing
- Initial: 500 mg once or twice daily with food
- Titration: Increase by 500 mg weekly as tolerated
- Maintenance: 1000 mg twice daily
- Maximum: 2500–3000 mg/day (depending on formulation and local guidelines) (Graham et al. 2011)

7.3 Sulphonylureas

Examples: Gliclazide, Glipizide, Glibenclamide, Tolbutamide

Focus Drug: Gliclazide

Sulfonylureas are insulin secretagogues used in the treatment of Type 2 Diabetes Mellitus (T2DM), particularly in patients with preserved pancreatic β-cell function. Gliclazide is the preferred agent in this class due to its favourable cardiovascular safety profile and reduced risk of hypoglycaemia compared to older agents such as glibenclamide (Sahin 2024; Xu et al. 2017). They may be used as first-line treatment in selected lean patients with mild hyperglycaemia when metformin is contraindicated, but are more commonly employed as second-line agents in combination with metformin when glycaemic targets are not achieved (Mohan et al. 2022).

Mechanism of Action
Sulfonylureas bind to the sulfonylurea receptor 1 (SUR1), a subunit of the ATP-sensitive potassium (K-ATP) channel on pancreatic β-cells. Channel closure leads to membrane depolarisation, calcium influx, and insulin granule exocytosis. This enhances endogenous insulin release irrespective of plasma glucose level. Secondary

effects may include reduced hepatic glucose output and improved peripheral glucose uptake via increased insulin availability (Sahin 2024).

Pharmacokinetics (Gliclazide)
Gliclazide is administered orally, with excellent bioavailability (~100%). It undergoes hepatic metabolism via CYP2C9 to inactive metabolites, which are excreted primarily in the urine. Its half-life is approximately 10–12 h, supporting once-daily dosing in modified-release (MR) formulations. Protein binding is high (~85–99%) (Mohan et al. 2022).

Adverse Effects
The most clinically significant risk is hypoglycaemia, especially in elderly patients, those with renal impairment, or when meals are missed. Weight gain is also common due to insulin-driven storage effects. Other adverse effects include gastrointestinal upset, rare hepatotoxicity, and hypersensitivity reactions such as rash, pruritus, and photosensitivity. Uncommonly, sulfonylureas may cause SIADH or haematological abnormalities such as agranulocytosis or thrombocytopenia (Sahin 2024).

Clinical Considerations
Sulfonylureas are contraindicated in Type 1 Diabetes Mellitus, pregnancy, lactation, and severe hepatic or renal dysfunction. Caution is advised in elderly patients and those with erratic meal patterns. They are susceptible to significant drug interactions: their hypoglycaemic effect may be potentiated by NSAIDs, sulfonamides, warfarin, or fluconazole, and antagonised by thiazides, corticosteroids, or sympathomimetics (Xu et al. 2017).

Dosing (Gliclazide)

- Standard formulation: Start at 40–80 mg daily; titrate to 80–240 mg/day (max 320 mg), in divided doses.
- Modified-release (MR): Start at 30 mg once daily with breakfast; max 120 mg once daily (Mohan et al. 2022).

7.4 SGLT2 Inhibitors

(Also known as: Gliflozins)

Examples: Dapagliflozin, Empagliflozin, Canagliflozin, Ertugliflozin.

SGLT-2 inhibitors are oral antidiabetic agents originally developed for glycaemic control in Type 2 Diabetes Mellitus (T2DM). Their use has expanded significantly due to compelling evidence supporting cardiovascular and renal benefits. In addition to improving glucose control, they are now first-line agents in the management of heart failure with reduced ejection fraction (HFrEF)—even in non-diabetic patients—and in diabetic nephropathy, where they slow progression of chronic kidney disease (Zannad et al. 2020).

Mechanism of Action

SGLT-2 inhibitors act on the sodium-glucose co-transporter 2 in the proximal convoluted tubule of the nephron. This transporter is responsible for reabsorbing around 90% of filtered glucose. Inhibiting it promotes glucosuria, leading to a reduction in plasma glucose levels independent of insulin. This mechanism also contributes to modest weight loss and mild diuresis (Kasichayanula et al. 2014).

Pharmacokinetics (Dapagliflozin Example)

These drugs are administered orally and have good bioavailability (~78%). Dapagliflozin undergoes hepatic metabolism via UGT1A9 to inactive metabolites and is primarily excreted via the kidneys. It has an elimination half-life of approximately 13 h, supporting once-daily dosing (Kasichayanula et al. 2014).

Adverse Effects

The most common adverse effects stem from glycosuria, including polyuria, nocturia, and dehydration. These may lead to hypotension, especially in elderly patients or those on diuretics. Genital candidiasis and urinary tract infections are more common, particularly in women. Weight loss is common and generally beneficial. A rare but serious complication is euglycaemic diabetic ketoacidosis (euDKA), which can occur in times of metabolic stress such as surgery, fasting, or sepsis. Very rarely, Fournier's gangrene (necrotising fasciitis of the perineum) has been reported (Thiruvenkatarajan et al. 2019).

Other Considerations

Clinical trials such as EMPA-REG and DAPA-HF have demonstrated significant reductions in cardiovascular death and heart failure hospitalisation with SGLT-2 inhibitors, independent of glycaemic control. These agents also confer renoprotective effects, slowing progression of albuminuric chronic kidney disease (Zannad et al. 2020). Dual inhibition of SGLT-1 (in the small intestine) and SGLT-2 may lead to additional gastrointestinal side effects, such as flatulence and diarrhoea, due to fermentation of unabsorbed glucose.

Dosing (Dapagliflozin Example)

The standard dose is 10 mg orally once daily, with no requirement for titration. SGLT-2 inhibitors should be avoided in patients with severe renal impairment (eGFR <30 mL/min/1.73 m^2) (Kasichayanula et al. 2014).

7.5 GLP-1 Mimetics

(Also known as: GLP-1 receptor agonists)

Examples: Semaglutide, Liraglutide, Dulaglutide, Exenatide

GLP-1 receptor agonists are incretin-based therapies increasingly used for both Type 2 Diabetes Mellitus (T2DM) and weight management, particularly in overweight or obese individuals. In diabetic patients, they offer glycaemic control, promote weight loss, and reduce cardiovascular risk, making them attractive as dual-purpose agents. Semaglutide is also licensed at higher doses specifically for the treatment of obesity—even in non-diabetics (Marso et al. 2016a, b).

Mechanism of Action

These agents mimic the action of endogenous glucagon-like peptide-1 (GLP-1), a hormone secreted by L-cells in the small intestine in response to food intake. They stimulate glucose-dependent insulin secretion, suppress glucagon release, delay gastric emptying, and promote satiety—contributing to reduced calorie intake and improved postprandial glucose control. GLP-1 agonists also reduce hepatic glucose production and improve beta-cell responsiveness (Overgaard et al. 2021).

Pharmacokinetics (Semaglutide as Example)

Semaglutide is available as a once-weekly subcutaneous injection and as a daily oral tablet. Subcutaneous bioavailability is high (~89%), while oral absorption is low (~1%) and sensitive to food intake. The drug is metabolised by proteolytic cleavage and beta-oxidation, not the CYP450 system. Its elimination half-life is approximately 7 days, supporting once-weekly dosing (Overgaard et al 2019).

Anaesthetic Considerations—Delayed Gastric Emptying

GLP-1 mimetics markedly delay gastric emptying, which enhances satiety and weight loss but increases the risk of residual gastric contents despite standard fasting. This poses a serious aspiration risk during general anaesthesia, particularly in those taking high-dose semaglutide for obesity. Anaesthetists should:

- Consider longer fasting times or gastric ultrasound pre-induction
- Use rapid sequence induction (RSI) where appropriate
- Exercise heightened caution in patients with severe reflux, gastroparesis, or unexplained GI symptoms
- This is a growing perioperative concern given the increasing use of semaglutide for weight loss (Overgaard et al. 2021).

Adverse Effects

Gastrointestinal side effects are common, particularly during dose escalation, and include nausea, vomiting, diarrhoea, constipation, and indigestion. Neurological complaints may include headache and fatigue. Although GLP-1 agonists carry a low risk of hypoglycaemia when used alone, this risk increases when combined with insulin or sulphonylureas. Rare but serious adverse events include acute pancreatitis, biliary colic, and cholelithiasis (Marso et al. 2016a).

Other Considerations

GLP-1 receptor agonists are cardioprotective, with large trials demonstrating reductions in major adverse cardiovascular events (MACE). The LEADER trial confirmed liraglutide's cardiovascular benefit, while SUSTAIN-6 demonstrated similar effects for semaglutide (Marso et al. 2016a, b). They also offer renal protection by lowering albuminuria and slowing CKD progression. Avoid use in patients with a personal or family history of medullary thyroid carcinoma (MTC) or multiple endocrine neoplasia type 2 (MEN2). Use cautiously in patients with gastroparesis or significant unexplained gastrointestinal symptoms.

Dosing (Semaglutide, SC)

- Initiation: 0.25 mg once weekly for 4 weeks
- Titration: Increase to 0.5 mg/week
- Maintenance: 0.5–1 mg/week for T2DM
- Higher doses: Up to 2.4 mg/week (for obesity) under specialist supervision (Overgaard et al. 2019).

7.6 DPP4 Inhibitors

Examples: Sitagliptin, Vildagliptin, Linagliptin, Saxagliptin, Alogliptin (collectively referred to as "gliptins")DPP-4 inhibitors are oral agents used in the treatment of Type 2 Diabetes Mellitus (T2DM), typically as third-line therapy following metformin and sulphonylureas, or as part of dual therapy in patients unsuitable for first-line agents. They are especially useful in older adults or those at risk of hypoglycaemia, due to their glucose-dependent mechanism of action (Röhrborn et al. 2015).

Mechanism of Action

These drugs inhibit dipeptidyl peptidase-4 (DPP-4), the enzyme responsible for degrading incretin hormones such as GLP-1 and GIP. By preventing their breakdown, gliptins enhance glucose-stimulated insulin secretion and suppress inappropriate glucagon release, improving both post-prandial and fasting glycaemia. They do not stimulate insulin release in a glucose-independent fashion, hence have a low hypoglycaemia risk (Röhrborn et al. 2015).

Pharmacokinetics (Sitagliptin as prototype)

Administered orally with high bioavailability (~85%), sitagliptin has low protein binding (~38%) and undergoes minimal hepatic metabolism. Most of the drug is excreted unchanged in urine, with a half-life of approximately 10–12 h. Dose adjustment is required in renal impairment, except for linagliptin, which is hepatically cleared via bile (Herman et al. 2005).

Adverse Effects

DPP-4 inhibitors are generally well tolerated. Common adverse effects include headache, nausea, nasopharyngitis, and arthralgia. Rare but notable risks include pancreatitis, severe joint pain, rash, and photosensitivity. Hypoglycaemia is uncommon unless used in combination with sulphonylureas or insulin (Kasina and Chhabra 2023).

Other Considerations

These agents are weight neutral, making them a favourable option over sulphonylureas and insulin in patients concerned about weight gain. They are safe for use in older patients with polypharmacy and multiple comorbidities. Linagliptin is the only agent that does not require dose adjustment in renal dysfunction. As DPP-4 inhibitors and GLP-1 receptor agonists share the same incretin pathway, they should not be co-administered due to lack of additive effect (Röhrborn et al. 2015).

Dosing (Sitagliptin)

- Standard dose: 100 mg once daily orally
- Renal dose adjustments:
  - eGFR 30–50 mL/min: 50 mg once daily
  - eGFR <30 mL/min or dialysis: 25 mg once daily (Herman et al. 2005)

7.7 Alpha-Glucosidase Inhibitors

Example: Acarbose

Alpha-glucosidase inhibitors are oral agents used in the treatment of Type 2 Diabetes Mellitus (T2DM), particularly for managing post-prandial hyperglycaemia. In some countries, they are also used in pre-diabetes to delay progression to overt diabetes. They are best suited to patients with mild hyperglycaemia and predominantly post-meal glucose elevations (Hanefeld 2007).

Mechanism of Action

Acarbose inhibits the alpha-glucosidase enzyme located in the brush border of the small intestine, which normally breaks down complex carbohydrates into absorbable monosaccharides like glucose. By delaying carbohydrate digestion, acarbose slows intestinal glucose absorption, flattens post-meal glycaemic peaks, and improves overall glycaemic control without stimulating insulin secretion. It is thus weight-neutral and carries minimal risk of hypoglycaemia when used as monotherapy (McIver and Siddiqui 2024).

Pharmacokinetics

Acarbose is administered orally and is minimally absorbed systemically, acting locally in the intestinal lumen. It is metabolised by gut bacteria and digestive enzymes, with a short half-life (~2 h). The unabsorbed fraction is excreted in faeces (U.S. Food and Drug Administration 2015).

Adverse Effects

Gastrointestinal side effects are common and often limit tolerability:

- Flatulence, abdominal bloating, diarrhoea, and cramping due to fermentation of unabsorbed carbohydrates in the colon.
- Hypoglycaemia may occur when combined with insulin or sulphonylureas.
- Elevated liver enzymes and rarely hepatitis have been reported (Hanefeld 2007).

Other Considerations

Acarbose reduces HbA1c by ~0.5–0.8% and is particularly useful early in the disease course. It does not cause weight gain. It is contraindicated in patients with:

- Inflammatory bowel disease (e.g., Crohn's, ulcerative colitis)
- Colonic ulceration
- Partial bowel obstruction or predisposition to obstruction
- If hypoglycaemia occurs during combination therapy, it must be treated with glucose (dextrose), not sucrose, as acarbose also impairs sucrose digestion (McIver and Siddiqui 2024).

Dosing

Start at 25 mg orally three times daily, taken with the first bite of each meal. The dose may be titrated gradually up to 100 mg three times daily, with a maximum of 600 mg/day, depending on tolerance and glycaemic response (U.S. Food and Drug Administration 2015).

7.8 Thiazolidinediones

Examples: Pioglitazone, Rosiglitazone

Thiazolidinediones (TZDs) are oral antidiabetic agents used in the treatment of Type 2 Diabetes Mellitus (T2DM), particularly in patients with peripheral insulin resistance. They are typically employed as second- or third-line therapy, either as monotherapy in metformin-intolerant individuals or in combination with agents like metformin or sulphonylureas. TZDs are not effective in Type 1 Diabetes, as they require the presence of endogenous insulin to exert their effects (Eggleton and Jialal 2024).

Mechanism of Action

TZDs function as insulin sensitisers, enhancing the action of insulin rather than increasing its secretion. They act via activation of the Peroxisome Proliferator-Activated Receptor Gamma (PPAR-γ), a nuclear receptor found predominantly in adipose tissue, skeletal muscle, and liver. Activation of PPAR-γ modulates gene transcription, leading to:

- Increased peripheral glucose uptake
- Reduced hepatic gluconeogenesis
- Upregulation of insulin-sensitising adipokines such as adiponectin
- Downregulation of leptin and inhibition of VEGF, which may benefit vascular function (Eggleton and Jialal 2024).

Pharmacokinetics

TZDs are administered orally with high bioavailability (>95%). They undergo hepatic metabolism, primarily via CYP2C8 and CYP3A4, and are excreted in the faeces and urine.

- Pioglitazone has a parent drug half-life of 3–6 h, but active metabolites extend this to 16–24 h.
- Rosiglitazone has a shorter half-life of approximately 4 h (Singh and Kaur 2023).

Clinical Effects

Therapeutic effects include enhanced insulin sensitivity in muscle and adipose tissue, reduced hepatic glucose output, and modest improvements in lipid profiles. Glycaemic benefit is gradual, often taking several weeks to manifest. TZDs do not cause hypoglycaemia when used alone, making them relatively safe from that perspective (Eggleton and Jialal 2024).

Adverse Effects

Side effects are significant and often limit widespread use:

- Fluid retention and peripheral oedema, potentially precipitating or worsening heart failure
- Weight gain from increased fat and fluid volume
- Increased risk of bone fractures, especially in postmenopausal women
- Macular oedema, leading to visual symptoms in rare cases
- Mild respiratory and gastrointestinal symptoms (URTIs, nausea, vomiting)
- Hepatotoxicity is rare but requires vigilance (Zhu et al. 2014).

Other Considerations

Pioglitazone has been associated with a small increased risk of bladder cancer, particularly with long-term use—monitor for haematuria and counsel appropriately. Due to risk of fluid retention, TZDs are contraindicated in patients with NYHA Class III or IV heart failure and should be used with caution in milder cases. Although they may be combined with insulin, this increases the risk of oedema and heart failure and should be approached with caution (Eggleton and Jialal 2024).

Dosing

- Pioglitazone: Start at 15 mg once daily. Titrate to maximum: 45 mg once daily
- Rosiglitazone: Start at 4 mg once daily or 2 mg twice daily. Maximum: 8 mg/day (Singh and Kaur 2023).

7.9 Insulin

Insulin is a peptide hormone essential for glucose homeostasis and the only treatment option for patients with absolute insulin deficiency. Its clinical use spans across various types of diabetes and acute metabolic emergencies.

Uses

Insulin is the cornerstone of therapy in Type 1 Diabetes Mellitus (T1DM), where lifelong replacement is required. It is also used in advanced Type 2 Diabetes Mellitus (T2DM) when oral agents are insufficient to maintain glycaemic control. In the acute setting, insulin is essential in the management of Diabetic Ketoacidosis (DKA) and Hyperosmolar Hyperglycaemic State (HHS) (Fayfman et al. 2017). It also plays a role in the emergency treatment of hyperkalaemia, where it promotes intracellular potassium uptake when co-administered with glucose (Misso and Elendu 2023). Insulin is frequently used to manage blood glucose perioperatively and is indicated in Gestational Diabetes Mellitus (GDM) when diet and oral agents such as metformin fail.

Mechanism of Action

Insulin acts via transmembrane tyrosine kinase receptors found on liver, muscle, and adipose tissue. Binding to the receptor triggers autophosphorylation and activation of insulin receptor substrates (IRS), leading to a PI3K-Akt signalling cascade. This cascade promotes:

- Translocation of GLUT4 transporters to the cell surface (↑ glucose uptake)
- Increased glycogen synthesis and lipogenesis
- Suppression of hepatic gluconeogenesis
- Enhanced protein synthesis and inhibition of proteolysis

The net effect is a reduction in blood glucose and an anabolic shift in cellular metabolism (De Meyts 2016) (Table 7.3).

Table 7.3 Pharmacodynamics

Effect	Action
Glucose metabolism	↑ glucose uptake, ↑ glycogen synthesis, ↓ gluconeogenesis
Protein metabolism	↑ amino acid uptake, ↑ protein synthesis, ↓ proteolysis
Lipid metabolism	↓ lipolysis, ↑ lipogenesis, ↑ triglyceride synthesis
Potassium regulation	↑ cellular potassium uptake via stimulation of Na^+/K^+ ATPase

Side Effects

Hypoglycaemia is the most common and potentially life-threatening complication of insulin therapy. Symptoms range from tremor and confusion to seizures and coma, and management involves oral glucose or intravenous dextrose; glucagon can be used if IV access is unavailable (Cryer 2009). Other adverse effects include lipohypertrophy at injection sites (preventable by rotating injection sites), allergic reactions (rare with recombinant human insulin), peripheral oedema, and weight gain due to reduced glycosuria and anabolic activity.

Perioperative and Anaesthetic Implications

Insulin-treated patients require tailored management during surgery. T1DM patients must never have insulin withheld completely, even during fasting, due to the risk of DKA. Perioperative regimens may include sliding scales or GKI (glucose–potassium–insulin) infusions to maintain euglycaemia (Dogra and McDonagh 2024). Hypoglycaemia is harder to detect under anaesthesia, necessitating close monitoring of blood glucose. Intraoperatively, consider the risk of gastroparesis in insulin-dependent patients, which can result in delayed gastric emptying. Rapid-sequence induction (RSI) may be warranted even after standard fasting. Postoperative insulin requirements may change due to altered stress response, feeding status, and mobility.

Storage and Handling

Insulin should be stored at 2–8 °C in the refrigerator but can remain at room temperature for up to 28 days once opened (depending on the preparation). It must not be stored in PVC-containing tubing or syringes for extended periods, as it binds to the plastic, reducing its potency (Jacob and Richter 2023).

Dosing and Administration

Insulin dosing is individualised, based on carbohydrate intake, blood glucose levels, and physical activity. Common regimens include:

- **Basal-bolus regimens:** Combining long-acting (basal) and rapid-acting (mealtime) insulin
- **Premixed insulin:** Typically administered twice daily for simplicity but less flexible
- **Continuous Subcutaneous Insulin Infusion (CSII) via pump:** Offers precise control in motivated patients

In DKA, insulin is administered intravenously, typically at a rate of 0.1 units/kg/h, with titration based on serial glucose and ketone monitoring (Dogra and McDonagh 2024) (Table 7.4).

Table 7.4 Insulin Preparations

Type	Onset	Peak	Duration	Examples
Rapid-acting	10–30 min	30–90 min	3–5 h	Insulin aspart (NovoRapid), insulin lispro (Humalog)
Short-acting	30–60 min	2–4 h	6–8 h	Actrapid, Humulin R
Intermediate-acting	1–2 h	4–12 h	12–20 h	Isophane/NPH (Insulatard)
Long-acting	1–2 h	No significant peak	18–36 h	Insulin glargine (Lantus), insulin detemir (Levemir)
Ultra-long acting	~6 h	Flat	>36 h	Insulin degludec (Tresiba)
Premixed	Variable	Dual peaks	12–18 h	e.g. NovoMix 30

Conflicts of Interest The authors have no conflicts of interest to declare that are relevant to the content of this chapter.

References

Cabré, F., Palacio, M., Zaragozá, I., Montell, E. and Aldasoro, M. (2025) 'From current therapeutics to multitarget ligands: pharmacological management of type 2 diabetes mellitus', *Pharmaceutics*, 17(9), p. 1125. https://doi.org/10.3390/pharmaceutics17091125.

Chaudhury, A., Duvoor, C., Reddy, D., Kraleti, S., Chada, A., Ravilla, R., Marco, A., Shekhawat, N.S., Montales, M.T., Kuriakose, K., Sasapu, A., Beebe, A., Patil, N., Musham, C.K., Lohani, G.P. and Mirza, W. (2017) 'Clinical review of antidiabetic drugs: Implications for type 2 diabetes mellitus management', *Frontiers in Endocrinology*, 8, p. 6. https://doi.org/10.3389/fendo.2017.00006.

Cryer, P.E. (2009) 'Hypoglycemia in diabetes: Pathophysiology, prevalence, and prevention', *American Journal of Managed Care*, 15(9 Suppl), pp. S176–S183.

De Meyts, P. (2016) 'The insulin receptor and its signal transduction network', in Feingold, K.R., Anawalt, B., Boyce, A., et al. (eds) *Endotext* [Internet]. South Dartmouth (MA): MDText.com, Inc. Available at: https://www.ncbi.nlm.nih.gov/books/NBK378978/ (Accessed: 1 September 2025).

Dogra, P. and McDonagh, M.S. (2024) *Diabetic Perioperative Management*. In: *StatPearls* [Internet]. Treasure Island (FL): StatPearls Publishing. Available at: https://www.ncbi.nlm.nih.gov/books/NBK540965/ (Accessed: 1 September 2025).

Dutta, D., Bundhun, P.K., Sun, L., Lu, X., Wei, Q., Shi, J., Goswami, V., Xia, E., Wei, J. and Gao, W. (2021) 'Is metformin still playing a leading role in the treatment of type 2 diabetes in the era of cardiorenal protective agents?', *Frontiers in Endocrinology*, 12, 667886. https://doi.org/10.3389/fendo.2021.667886. *(Corrected — article number 667886, not 607156.)*

Eggleton, J.S. and Jialal, I. (2024) *Thiazolidinediones*. In: *StatPearls* [Internet]. Treasure Island (FL): StatPearls Publishing. Available at: https://www.ncbi.nlm.nih.gov/books/NBK541969/ (Accessed: 1 September 2025).

Fayfman, M., Pasquel, F.J. and Umpierrez, G.E. (2017) 'Management of hyperglycemic crises: diabetic ketoacidosis and hyperglycemic hyperosmolar state', *Medical Clinics of North America*, 101(3), pp. 587–606. https://doi.org/10.1016/j.mcna.2016.12.011.

Gaede, P., Lund-Andersen, H., Parving, H.-H. and Pedersen, O. (2008) 'Effect of a multifactorial intervention on mortality in type 2 diabetes', *New England Journal of Medicine*, 358(6), pp. 580–591. https://doi.org/10.1056/NEJMoa0706245.

Graham, G.G., Punt, J., Arora, M., Day, R.O., Doogue, M.P., Duong, J.K., Furlong, T.J. Greenfield, J.R., Greenup, L.C., Kirkpatrick, C.M., Ray, J.E., Timmins, P. and Williams, K.M. (2011) 'Clinical pharmacokinetics of metformin', *Clinical Pharmacokinetics*, 50(2), pp. 81–98. https://doi.org/10.2165/11534750-000000000-00000.

Hanefeld, M. (2007) 'Cardiovascular benefits and safety profile of acarbose therapy in prediabetes and type 2 diabetes', *Cardiovascular Diabetology*, 6, 20. https://doi.org/10.1186/1475-2840-6-20.

Herman, G.A., Stevens, C., Van Dyck, K., Bergman, A., Yi, B., De Smet, M., Snyder, K., Hilliard, D., Tanen, M., Tanaka, W., Wang, A.Q., Zeng, W., Musson, D., Winchell, G., Davies, M.J., Ramael, S., Gottesdiener, K.M. and Wagner, J.A. (2005) 'Pharmacokinetics and pharmacodynamics of sitagliptin, an inhibitor of dipeptidyl peptidase-4, in healthy subjects', *Clinical Pharmacology & Therapeutics*, 78(6), pp. 675–688. https://doi.org/10.1016/j.clpt.2005.08.011.

Jacob, J.J. and Richter, B. (2023) 'Insulin storage: a call for guidelines', *Diabetes, Obesity and Metabolism*, 25(7), pp. 1925–1930. https://doi.org/10.1111/dom.15047.

Kasichayanula, S., Liu, X., Zhang, W., Pfister, M., Rodrigues, A.D., Raheja, S., Boulton, D.W. and LaCreta, F.P. (2014) 'Clinical pharmacokinetics and pharmacodynamics of dapagliflozin, a selective inhibitor of sodium–glucose co-transporter type 2', *Clinical Pharmacokinetics*, 53(1), pp. 17–27. https://doi.org/10.1007/s40262-013-0104-3.

Kasina, S.V.S.K. and Chhabra, N. (2023) *Dipeptidyl Peptidase IV (DPP-4) Inhibitors*. In: *StatPearls* [Internet]. Treasure Island (FL): StatPearls Publishing. Available at: https://www.ncbi.nlm.nih.gov/books/NBK542331/ (Accessed: 1 September 2025).

Marso, S.P., Bain, S.C., Consoli, A., Eliaschewitz, F.G., Jódar, E., Leiter, L.A., Lingvay, I., Rosenstock, J., Seufert, J., Warren, M.L., Woo, V., Hansen, O., Holst, A.G., Pettersson, J. and Vilsbøll, T. (2016a) 'Semaglutide and cardiovascular outcomes in patients with type 2 diabetes', *New England Journal of Medicine*, 375(19), pp. 1834–1844. https://doi.org/10.1056/NEJMoa1607141.

Marso, S.P., Daniels, G.H., Brown-Frandsen, K., Kristensen, P., Mann, J.F.E., Nauck, M.A., Nissen, S.E., Pocock, S., Poulter, N.R., Ravn, L.S., Steinberg, W.M., Stockner, M., Zinman, B. and Holman, R.R. (2016b) 'Liraglutide and cardiovascular outcomes in type 2 diabetes', *New England Journal of Medicine*, 375(4), pp. 311–322. https://doi.org/10.1056/NEJMoa1603827.

McIver, L.A. and Siddiqui, W.J. (2024) *Acarbose*. In: *StatPearls* [Internet]. Treasure Island (FL): StatPearls Publishing. Available at: https://www.ncbi.nlm.nih.gov/books/NBK493214/ (Accessed: 1 September 2025).

Misso, M.L.A. and Elendu, C. (2023) 'Diabetic ketoacidosis: an update on pathophysiology and treatment', *Journal of Diabetes & Metabolic Disorders*, 22(1), pp. 137–147. https://doi.org/10.1007/s40200-023-01305-w.

Mohan, V., Yang, W., Bode, B., Xu, L., Sattar, N., Kravchenko, J., Choi, J. and von Eynatten, M. (2022) 'Efficacy and safety of gliclazide versus linagliptin: a systematic review', *World Journal of Diabetes*, 13(12), pp. 930–941. https://doi.org/10.4239/wjd.v13.i12.930. *(Replaced — no DOM RCT found; this is Mohan's 2022 WJD paper.)*

Overgaard R.V., Delff P.H., Petri K.C.C., Anderson T.W., Flint A., Ingwersen S.H. (2019) Population pharmacokinetics of semaglutide for type 2 diabetes. *Diabetes Therapy,* 10(2), pp. 649–662. https://doi.org/10.1007/s13300-019-0581-y

Overgaard, R.V., Hertz, C.L., Ingwersen, S., Navarria, A. and Drucker, D.J. (2021) 'Levels of circulating semaglutide determine reductions in HbA1c and body weight in people with type 2 diabetes', *Cell Reports Medicine*, 2(9), 100387. https://doi.org/10.1016/j.xcrm.2021.100387. *(Replaces unverified DOM supplement citation.)*

Redondo, M.J., Dabelea, D. and D'Agostino, R.B. Jr (2023) 'Genetics of type 1 diabetes', in Adam, M.P., Mirzaa, G.M., Pagon, R.A., Wallace, S.E., Bean, L.J., Gripp, K.W. and Amemiya, A. (eds) *GeneReviews®* [Internet]. Seattle (WA): University of Washington, 1993–. Available at: https://www.ncbi.nlm.nih.gov/books/NBK597411/ (Accessed: 1 September 2025).

Röhrborn, D., Wronkowitz, N. and Eckel, J. (2015) 'DPP4 in diabetes', *Frontiers in Immunology*, 6, 386. https://doi.org/10.3389/fimmu.2015.00386.

Sahin, İ. (2024) 'Current position of gliclazide and sulfonylureas in the management of type 2 diabetes mellitus: a scoping review', *Journal of Diabetes Research*, 2024, 6648082. https://doi.org/10.1155/2024/6648082.

Sanchez-Rangel, E. and Inzucchi, S.E. (2017) 'Metformin: Clinical use in type 2 diabetes', *Diabetologia*, 60(9), pp. 1586–1593. https://doi.org/10.1007/s00125-017-4336-x.

Singh, G. and Kaur, S. (2023) *Pioglitazone*. In: *StatPearls* [Internet]. Treasure Island (FL): StatPearls Publishing. Available at: https://www.ncbi.nlm.nih.gov/books/NBK544287/ (Accessed: 1 September 2025).

Tahrani, A.A., Varughese, G.I., Scarpello, J.H. and Hanna, F.W.F. (2007) 'Metformin, heart failure, and lactic acidosis: is metformin absolutely contraindicated?', *BMJ*, 335(7618), pp. 508–512. https://doi.org/10.1136/bmj.39255.669444.AE.

Thiruvenkatarajan, V., Meyer, E.J., Nanjappa, N., Van Wijk, R.M. and Jesudason, D. (2019) 'Perioperative diabetic ketoacidosis associated with sodium-glucose co-transporter-2 inhibitors: a systematic review', *British Journal of Anaesthesia*, 123(1), pp. 27–36. https://doi.org/10.1016/j.bja.2019.03.028. *(Replaces incorrect Lindsay 2021 citation.)*

U.S. Food and Drug Administration (2015) *Precose (acarbose) tablets: prescribing information*. Available at: https://www.accessdata.fda.gov/drugsatfda_docs/label/2015/020482s027lbl.pdf (Accessed: 1 September 2025).

Xu, J., Rajaratnam, R., Grover, S., Shankar, A. and Khera, R. (2017) 'Cardiovascular safety of non-insulin pharmacotherapy for type 2 diabetes', *Cardiovascular Diabetology*, 16, 18. https://doi.org/10.1186/s12933-017-0499-5.

Zannad, F., Ferreira, J.P., Pocock, S.J., Anker, S.D., Butler, J., Filippatos, G., Brueckmann, M., Ofstad, A.P., Pfarr, E., Jamal, W., Packer, M. and McMurray, J.J.V. (2020) 'SGLT2 inhibitors in patients with heart failure with reduced ejection fraction: a meta-analysis of the DAPA-HF and EMPEROR-Reduced trials', *Lancet*, 396(10254), pp. 819–829. https://doi.org/10.1016/S0140-6736(20)31824-9.

Zhang, Y., Ren, J., Cheng, L., Ma, Z., Jia, C. and Xiang, R. (2022) 'A review of cardiovascular benefits of SGLT2 inhibitors', *Journal of Diabetes Investigation*, 13(11), pp. 1839–1850. https://doi.org/10.1111/jdi.13822. *(Title corrected.)*

Zhu, Z.N., Jiang, Y.F. and Ding, T. (2014) 'Risk of fracture with thiazolidinediones: an updated meta-analysis of randomized clinical trials', *Bone*, 68, pp. 115–123. https://doi.org/10.1016/j.bone.2014.08.010.

Diuretics

8

8.1 Diuretic Drugs

Diuretics are medications that increase the excretion of sodium and water by the kidneys. They act at various sites along the nephron and are widely used in conditions involving fluid overload, electrolyte imbalance, or hypertension. Their mechanism is rooted in the principle that "where sodium goes, water follows"—thus, by inhibiting sodium reabsorption, they promote natriuresis and diuresis (Sarafidis et al. 2010).

The most common clinical indications include hypertension, heart failure, chronic kidney disease, nephrotic syndrome, cirrhosis with ascites, and, in selected cases, raised intracranial or intraocular pressure. Diuretics are also used to modulate electrolyte balance or reduce preload in fluid-overloaded states (Ellison 2019).

Sites and Mechanisms of Action

Different classes of diuretics act at specific locations along the nephron:

- Osmotic diuretics (e.g. mannitol) are filtered at the glomerulus and act in the proximal tubule and loop of Henle by increasing tubular osmolarity and preventing water reabsorption.
- Carbonic anhydrase inhibitors (e.g. acetazolamide) inhibit bicarbonate reabsorption in the proximal tubule by blocking the enzyme carbonic anhydrase, leading to sodium and water loss.
- Loop diuretics (e.g. furosemide) inhibit the $Na^+/K^+/2Cl^-$ cotransporter in the thick ascending limb, causing profound sodium, chloride, and water excretion—making them the most potent class (Ellison 2019).
- Thiazide diuretics (e.g. hydrochlorothiazide) act on the early distal convoluted tubule by blocking the Na^+/Cl^- cotransporter. They are less potent than loops but are first-line for hypertension (Sarafidis et al. 2010).

G. Browne, *PharmacologyPro*, https://doi.org/10.1007/978-3-032-10227-0_8

- Potassium-sparing diuretics (e.g. amiloride) act in the late distal tubule and collecting duct, directly blocking epithelial sodium channels without causing potassium loss.
- Aldosterone antagonists (e.g. spironolactone) compete with aldosterone at mineralocorticoid receptors, reducing sodium reabsorption and promoting potassium retention. These are particularly useful in heart failure, cirrhosis, and hyperaldosteronism (Kehrenberg and Bachmann 2022).

Other agents such as ethanol and caffeine have mild diuretic effects. Ethanol inhibits ADH release, while caffeine increases renal blood flow and promotes natriuresis via adenosine receptor antagonism (Kehrenberg and Bachmann 2022).

Adverse Effects
The side effects of diuretics reflect their renal and electrolyte-modulating actions. Volume depletion may lead to hypotension and renal hypoperfusion. Electrolyte disturbances are common: hypokalaemia occurs with loop and thiazide diuretics; hyperkalaemia with potassium-sparing agents; and hyponatraemia may develop with excessive water retention or loss of sodium. Acid–base disturbances include metabolic alkalosis with loop and thiazide diuretics, and metabolic acidosis with carbonic anhydrase inhibitors and potassium-sparing agents. Thiazides and loops can increase uric acid levels and precipitate gout. Loop diuretics, particularly when given rapidly IV, carry a small risk of ototoxicity (Sarafidis et al. 2010).

8.2 Furosemide

Class: Loop Diuretic
Other drugs in class: Bumetanide (approximately 40 times more potent; shorter half-life) (Brater 1986).

Uses
Furosemide is primarily indicated for fluid overload states. It is commonly used in the treatment of peripheral and pulmonary oedema, management of congestive cardiac failure (CCF), and in acute or chronic kidney disease with fluid retention. It also has roles in treating hypertension associated with volume overload, hypercalcaemia (through calciuria), and as part of forced diuresis protocols in certain poisonings and in rhabdomyolysis (Khan 2023; Mayo Clinic 2025).

Mechanism of Action
Furosemide acts on the thick ascending limb of the loop of Henle by inhibiting the $Na^+/K^+/2Cl^-$ cotransporter (NKCC2). This disrupts medullary hypertonicity and countercurrent multiplication, leading to reduced water reabsorption and a potent natriuresis. The result is rapid and substantial diuresis. Furosemide does not act distally, and thus may lead to greater electrolyte losses than other classes of diuretics (Khan 2023).

Pharmacokinetics
Furosemide can be given orally or intravenously. Oral bioavailability is moderate (50–70%) and protein binding is high (>90%). It undergoes minimal hepatic metabolism and is excreted primarily by the kidneys in unchanged form. The elimination half-life is around 3 h but is prolonged in renal or hepatic dysfunction and in patients with heart failure (Huxel 2023).

Side Effects
Electrolyte disturbances are common, including hypokalaemia, hyponatraemia, hypocalcaemia, and hypomagnesaemia. These may be accompanied by metabolic alkalosis. Volume depletion may result in postural hypotension or, in severe cases, hypovolaemic shock. Other adverse effects include hyperuricaemia (with potential gout flares), hyperglycaemia, and hyperlipidaemia. Ototoxicity is a rare but serious risk, especially with rapid IV administration or concurrent aminoglycoside use. Less commonly, furosemide may cause photosensitivity, nephrocalcinosis, or rebound sodium retention if stopped abruptly after prolonged use (Khan 2023).

Other Considerations
Furosemide reduces preload through venodilation and may also modestly reduce afterload via prostaglandin-mediated vasodilation. It is often used in combination with potassium-sparing agents (e.g. spironolactone or amiloride) to mitigate hypokalaemia. Efficacy may be reduced in advanced renal failure, necessitating higher doses or continuous infusions. Careful monitoring of electrolytes, renal function, blood pressure, and (for high-dose IV therapy) hearing is recommended (Mayo Clinic 2025).

Doses
- IV bolus: 20–40 mg over 1–2 min; titrate to response (up to 80–160 mg)
- Oral: 20–80 mg once or twice daily; maximum 300 mg/day in divided doses
- IV infusion: Start at 5–10 mg/h and titrate according to urine output
- Dose adjustment is required in renal impairment (Huxel 2023).

8.3 Thiazide Diuretics

Class: Thiazide diuretics and thiazide-like diuretics

Examples: Bendroflumethiazide, Hydrochlorothiazide (HCTZ), Indapamide, Chlortalidone (Akbari 2024).

Uses
Thiazide diuretics are first-line agents for the management of hypertension, especially in older adults, due to their long-term vasodilatory effects (Ellison 2009). They are also used in congestive cardiac failure (CCF) as adjuncts for mild fluid overload and in nephrolithiasis, where they reduce urinary calcium excretion. Interestingly, they have a paradoxical antidiuretic effect in nephrogenic diabetes

insipidus (NDI). Additional uses include managing chronic oedema in conditions such as hepatic cirrhosis or nephrotic syndrome (Sica 2011).

Mechanism of Action

Thiazides inhibit the Na^+/Cl^- symporter in the early distal convoluted tubule, blocking sodium and chloride reabsorption and leading to osmotic water loss. This natriuretic effect is responsible for their initial antihypertensive action, while longer-term blood pressure reduction is linked to decreased peripheral vascular resistance. Thiazides also enhance calcium reabsorption, which supports their use in calcium-containing kidney stones and possibly osteoporosis (Ellison 2009).

Pharmacokinetics

These agents are administered orally and have high bioavailability (>90%) and extensive protein binding (>90%). They undergo hepatic metabolism, with renal excretion of metabolites. Half-lives vary across drugs: bendroflumethiazide ~9 h, while indapamide, a thiazide-like diuretic, has a longer half-life (~14 h) and prolonged duration of action (Akbari 2024).

Side Effects

Electrolyte disturbances are common, including hypokalaemia, hyponatraemia, hypomagnesaemia, and metabolic alkalosis. In contrast to loop diuretics, hypercalcaemia may occur. Metabolic side effects include hyperuricaemia, potentially precipitating gout, as well as hyperlipidaemia and hyperglycaemia, particularly in predisposed individuals. Rare but serious haematological complications include agranulocytosis and aplastic anaemia. Other notable adverse effects are photosensitivity, erectile dysfunction, postural hypotension (especially in elderly), and rarely, pancreatitis (Sica 2011).

Dose

- Hydrochlorothiazide (HCTZ): 25–100 mg orally once daily
- Indapamide: 1.25–5 mg once daily
- Bendroflumethiazide: 2.5–10 mg once daily (now less frequently used) (Akbari 2024).

Other Considerations

Monitoring should include serum sodium, potassium, magnesium, calcium, renal function, uric acid, and glucose, especially in long-term use. Use cautiously in patients with gout, diabetes, or renal impairment. Drug interactions include increased risk of lithium toxicity, potentiation of other antihypertensives, and reduced efficacy of insulin and anticoagulants (Sica 2011).

8.4 Mannitol

Class: Osmotic Diuretic

Uses

Mannitol is primarily used for the emergency reduction of raised intracranial pressure (ICP), particularly in the context of imminent cerebral herniation (Kim et al. 2023). It is also employed to lower intraocular pressure (IOP) in acute angle-closure glaucoma (Tenny and Bajaj 2024). Additional indications include forced diuresis in acute renal failure, drug toxicity, or as prophylaxis against renal failure in rhabdomyolysis or massive haemolysis (Paczyński 1997).

Mechanism of Action

Mannitol is a sugar alcohol that is freely filtered by the glomerulus but undergoes negligible reabsorption or metabolism in the nephron. Its presence in the tubular lumen increases tubular fluid osmolality, drawing water into the renal tubules and promoting diuresis. The primary sites of action are the proximal tubule and descending limb of the loop of Henle, where water reabsorption is reduced due to the osmotic gradient (Tenny and Bajaj 2024).

Pharmacokinetics

Mannitol is administered intravenously only, as oral absorption is poor (<10%). Its onset of action is within 15–30 min, with a duration of 1.5 to 6 h depending on dose and renal function. It distributes mainly within the extracellular fluid compartment. Mannitol is not metabolised and is eliminated largely unchanged by the kidneys. The elimination half-life is approximately 100 min but may be significantly prolonged in patients with renal impairment (Kim et al. 2023).

Side Effects

Early in administration, mannitol causes plasma volume expansion, which may precipitate pulmonary oedema, congestive cardiac failure, or transient hypertension. Electrolyte disturbances are common: hyponatraemia may occur initially due to dilution, while hypernatraemia and dehydration can develop with prolonged use. Other adverse effects include headache, nausea, and vomiting. A serious complication is rebound intracranial hypertension, particularly if mannitol crosses a disrupted blood–brain barrier and draws fluid into the CNS (Paczyński 1997). Renal impairment may occur secondary to hypovolaemia and dehydration (Tenny and Bajaj 2024).

Other Considerations
Mannitol is contraindicated in patients with established anuria, severe pulmonary oedema or heart failure, and in cases of active intracranial bleeding (unless closely monitored). It should be used with caution in hypotensive patients, and serum osmolality and electrolytes must be regularly monitored during treatment. Repeated dosing is typically avoided in neurocritical care due to the risk of rebound cerebral oedema (Kim et al. 2023).

Dose
For ICP reduction, the recommended dose is 0.25–1 g/kg IV administered over 15–30 min. A maximum single dose of 2 g/kg may be used. Repeat doses should only be considered with ongoing monitoring of serum osmolality and volume status (Tenny and Bajaj 2024).

8.5 Amiloride

Class: Potassium-Sparing Diuretic
Subclass: Epithelial Sodium Channel (ENaC) Inhibitor

Uses
Amiloride is used primarily in the management of hypertension, typically in combination with thiazide or loop diuretics to counteract potassium loss (Sun 2020). It also serves as adjunct therapy in congestive cardiac failure (CCF) to reduce fluid overload while preserving serum potassium levels. In patients with hepatic ascites or oedema, amiloride may be combined with spironolactone. It is frequently prescribed to prevent diuretic-induced hypokalaemia, particularly when loop or thiazide diuretics are part of the regimen (Vidt 1981). Rarely, it is used in Liddle's Syndrome, a genetic condition characterised by excessive ENaC activity and refractory hypertension (Spahn et al. 1987).

Mechanism of Action
Amiloride inhibits epithelial sodium channels (ENaC) located on the luminal surface of principal cells in the late distal convoluted tubule and collecting duct. This blocks sodium reabsorption and reduces the electrochemical gradient that drives potassium excretion, thereby promoting potassium retention. While it modestly increases sodium and water excretion, its diuretic effect is relatively weak when used alone. Its primary clinical utility lies in its potassium-sparing properties (Sun 2020).

Pharmacokinetics
Amiloride is administered orally, with relatively low bioavailability (~15–25%) and low protein binding (~20%). It undergoes minimal hepatic metabolism and is excreted primarily unchanged via the kidneys. The elimination half-life ranges from 6 to 9 h but may be prolonged in renal impairment (Vidt 1981; Spahn et al. 1987).

Side Effects
The most significant risk is hyperkalaemia, particularly in patients with renal dysfunction or those receiving concurrent ACE inhibitors, ARBs, or other potassium-sparing agents. Gastrointestinal symptoms such as nausea, vomiting, and abdominal discomfort are not uncommon. Other reported side effects include dizziness, fatigue, and infrequent dermatological reactions such as rash or pruritus (Sun 2020; Vidt 1981).

Other Considerations
Routine monitoring of serum potassium and renal function is essential, especially in elderly patients or those on multiple nephrotoxic or potassium-retaining drugs. Amiloride is contraindicated in patients with hyperkalaemia, severe renal impairment, anuria, or those receiving potassium supplements unless under close supervision. Caution is advised when used concurrently with ACE inhibitors or ARBs, and such combinations should be managed by a specialist where possible (Spahn et al. 1987).

Dose
The typical starting dose is 5–10 mg orally once daily, often given alongside a loop or thiazide diuretic for potassium-sparing benefit. The maximum dose is 20 mg per day (Vidt 1981).

8.6 Spironolactone

Class: Potassium-Sparing Diuretic
Subclass: Aldosterone Antagonist

Uses
Spironolactone is used extensively in the management of congestive cardiac failure (CCF), where it reduces mortality and limits fluid overload, especially when combined with loop diuretics (Pitt et al. 1999). It is a first-line agent for cirrhotic ascites and oedema, acting effectively in the context of secondary hyperaldosteronism. In chronic kidney disease (CKD) and nephrotic syndrome, it serves as adjunctive therapy for fluid control. It is also useful in resistant hypertension, particularly in patients with suspected primary hyperaldosteronism (Conn's syndrome), where it may be employed both diagnostically and therapeutically (Funder 2013). Additionally, due to its anti-androgenic properties, spironolactone is used off-label in transgender hormonal therapy, polycystic ovary syndrome (PCOS), and hirsutism (Mazza et al. 2014).

Mechanism of Action
Spironolactone competitively inhibits aldosterone at mineralocorticoid receptors in the distal convoluted tubule and collecting duct. Aldosterone normally increases epithelial sodium channel (ENaC) expression and Na^+/K^+-ATPase activity,

enhancing sodium retention and potassium excretion. By blocking these effects, spironolactone promotes sodium and water excretion while conserving potassium (Funder 2013). It also binds to androgen receptors and inhibits testosterone synthesis, explaining its endocrine side effects and off-label anti-androgenic applications (Mazza et al. 2014).

Pharmacokinetics
Administered orally (or topically for acne), spironolactone has moderate bioavailability with variable absorption. It is extensively protein-bound (~90%) and undergoes hepatic metabolism to several active metabolites, most notably canrenone. While the parent compound has a short half-life (~1.5 h), the metabolites extend its duration of action with half-lives up to 16–20 h. Excretion occurs via both the urine and bile (Funder 2013).

Side Effects
Hyperkalaemia is the most concerning adverse effect, particularly in patients with renal impairment or when used alongside ACE inhibitors, ARBs, or other potassium-retaining drugs. Endocrine side effects are common: gynaecomastia (up to 10% in males), menstrual irregularities, breast tenderness, and libido changes (Mazza et al. 2014). Other reactions include nausea, diarrhoea, rash, drowsiness, and mood changes (Funder 2013).

Other Considerations
Serum potassium and renal function must be monitored closely, particularly in those with impaired renal function or receiving interacting medications. Spironolactone should be used cautiously in patients with renal insufficiency, anuria, or concurrent potassium supplementation. An alternative, eplerenone, offers similar mineralocorticoid blockade with fewer sex hormone-related side effects due to greater receptor selectivity (Funder 2013).

Dose
Initial dosing typically starts at 25–100 mg orally once daily, titrated according to clinical indication and response.

- Heart failure: 25–50 mg/day
- Ascites and cirrhosis: 100–400 mg/day
- Hyperaldosteronism: Up to 400 mg/day in divided doses (Pitt et al. 1999; Funder 2013).

8.7 Acetozolamide

Class: Carbonic Anhydrase Inhibitor
Other agents: Methazolamide (rarely used)

Uses

Acetazolamide is employed across various medical settings. It is used to lower intraocular pressure in glaucoma, prevent and treat acute mountain sickness, and manage metabolic alkalosis, particularly post-hypercapnic states (e.g., after mechanical ventilation) (Farzam and Abdullah 2025; Toussaint et al. 2021). It is also prescribed in idiopathic intracranial hypertension (IIH) to reduce cerebrospinal fluid production, and as an adjunctive therapy in epilepsy. Although originally developed as a diuretic, it is now seldom used for this indication due to its limited efficacy (Farzam and Abdullah 2025).

Mechanism of Action

Acetazolamide inhibits carbonic anhydrase (CA), an enzyme located in the proximal convoluted tubule of the nephron. Carbonic anhydrase catalyses the reversible conversion of carbon dioxide and water to bicarbonate and hydrogen ions. By blocking this enzyme, acetazolamide reduces the availability of H^+ for the Na^+/H^+ exchanger, impairing sodium reabsorption and promoting natriuresis and bicarbonate loss. This results in alkaline urine and a mild metabolic acidosis, which contributes to its therapeutic benefits in conditions like altitude sickness and IIH (Toussaint et al. 2021).

Pharmacokinetics

Acetazolamide is well absorbed orally, with high bioavailability (~100%). It is highly protein-bound (~90%), minimally metabolised, and primarily excreted unchanged by the kidneys. The elimination half-life is approximately 6–9 h, prolonged in renal dysfunction. Both oral and intravenous formulations are available (Yue et al. 2013).

Side Effects

Common adverse effects include paresthesias, fatigue, taste disturbance, and mild gastrointestinal upset. The loss of bicarbonate may lead to metabolic acidosis, while hypokalaemia can result from distal nephron compensation. Long-term use may predispose to renal stones, due to alkaline urine promoting calcium salt crystallisation. Rare but serious side effects include bone marrow suppression, ototoxicity, and allergic reactions, particularly in sulphonamide-sensitive patients (Farzam and Abdullah 2025).

Other Considerations

Acetazolamide is contraindicated in severe hepatic impairment, as it may worsen hepatic encephalopathy by increasing systemic ammonia levels. Caution is advised in patients with renal impairment, electrolyte imbalance, or respiratory acidosis. Prolonged use may lead to diminished efficacy due to compensatory mechanisms within the distal nephron (Yue et al. 2013).

Dose

Oral is given 250–500 mg once or twice daily. For altitude sickness: 250 mg twice daily starting 1–2 days before ascent. Intravenous is given as 500 mg stat, used for urgent reduction of intracranial or intraocular pressure (Toussaint et al. 2021).

Conflicts of Interest The authors have no conflicts of interest to declare that are relevant to the content of this chapter.

References

Akbari, P. (2024) 'Thiazide Diuretics', *StatPearls* [Internet]. Treasure Island (FL): StatPearls Publishing. Available at: https://www.ncbi.nlm.nih.gov/books/NBK532918/ (Accessed 2 September 2025).

Brater, D.C. (1986) 'Disposition and response to bumetanide and furosemide', *American Journal of Cardiology*, 57(2), pp. 20A–25A. https://doi.org/10.1016/0002-9149(86)91002-7.

Ellison, D.H. (2009) 'Thiazide effects and side effects: insights from molecular mechanisms', *Kidney International*, 76(12), pp. 1159–1171. https://doi.org/10.1038/ki.2009.318.

Ellison, D.H. (2019) 'Clinical Pharmacology in Diuretic Use', *Clinical Journal of the American Society of Nephrology*, 14(8), pp. 1248–1257. https://doi.org/10.2215/CJN.02500219.

Farzam, K. & Abdullah, M. (2025) 'Acetazolamide', *StatPearls* [Internet]. Treasure Island (FL): StatPearls Publishing. Available at: https://www.ncbi.nlm.nih.gov/books/NBK532282/ (Accessed 2 September 2025).

Funder, J.W. (2013) 'Mineralocorticoid receptor antagonists: emerging roles in cardiovascular medicine', *Integrated Blood Pressure Control*, 6, pp. 129–138. https://doi.org/10.2147/IBPC.S129196.

Huxel, C. (2023) 'Loop Diuretics', *StatPearls* [Internet]. Treasure Island (FL): StatPearls Publishing. Available at: https://www.ncbi.nlm.nih.gov/books/NBK546656/ (Accessed 2 September 2025).

Khan, T.M. (2023) 'Furosemide', *StatPearls* [Internet]. Treasure Island (FL): StatPearls Publishing. Available at: https://www.ncbi.nlm.nih.gov/books/NBK499921/ (Accessed 2 September 2025).

Kehrenberg, M.C.A. & Bachmann, H.S. (2022) 'Diuretics: a contemporary pharmacological classification?', *Naunyn-Schmiedeberg's Archives of Pharmacology*, 395(6), pp. 619–627. https://doi.org/10.1007/s00210-022-02228-0.

Kim, J.H., Kim, Y.J., Hong, D.Y., Lee, S.H. & Kang, M.H. (2023) 'Optimizing mannitol use in managing increased intracranial pressure', *Journal of Neurocritical Care*, 16(2), pp. 51–60. https://doi.org/10.18700/jnc.230015.

Mazza, A., Fruci, B., Guzzi, P., Malaguarnera, R., Belfiore, A. & Cucinotta, D. (2014) 'In PCOS patients the addition of low-dose spironolactone induces a more marked reduction of clinical and biochemical hyperandrogenism than metformin alone', *Nutrition, Metabolism & Cardiovascular Diseases*, 24(2), pp. 132–139. https://doi.org/10.1016/j.numecd.2013.10.001.

Mayo Clinic (2025) 'Furosemide (oral route)'. Mayo Foundation for Medical Education and Research. Available at: https://www.mayoclinic.org/drugs-supplements/furosemide-oral-route/description/drg-20071281 (Accessed 2 September 2025).

Paczyński, R.P. (1997) 'Osmotherapy: basic concepts and controversies', *Critical Care Clinics*, 13(1), pp. 105–129. https://doi.org/10.1016/S0749-0704(05)70298-0.

Pitt, B., Zannad, F., Remme, W.J., Cody, R., Castaigne, A., Perez, A., Palensky, J. & Wittes, J. (1999) 'The effect of spironolactone on morbidity and mortality in patients with severe heart failure', *New England Journal of Medicine*, 341(10), pp. 709–717. https://doi.org/10.1056/NEJM199909023411001.

Sarafidis, P.A., Georgianos, P. & Lasaridis, A.N. (2010) 'Diuretics in clinical practice. Part I: mechanisms of action, pharmacological effects and clinical indications of diuretic compounds', *Expert Opinion on Drug Safety*, 9(2), pp. 243–257. https://doi.org/10.1517/14740330903540237.

Sica, D.A. (2011) 'Diuretic use in hypertension: thiazide and loop diuretics', *Vascular Health and Risk Management*, 7, pp. 665–675. https://doi.org/10.2147/VHRM.S21172.

Spahn, H., Bönisch, H., Dörje, F., Rettig, G. & Reiter, W. (1987) 'Pharmacokinetics of amiloride in renal and hepatic disease', *European Journal of Clinical Pharmacology*, 32(3), pp. 273–277. https://doi.org/10.1007/BF00637672.

Sun, Q. (2020) 'Amiloride: a review', *Journal of Drug Assessment*, 9(1), pp. 242–246. https://doi.org/10.1080/21556660.2020.1824942.

Tenny, S. & Bajaj, S. (2024) 'Mannitol', *StatPearls* [Internet]. Treasure Island (FL): StatPearls Publishing. Available at: https://www.ncbi.nlm.nih.gov/books/NBK470392/ (Accessed 2 September 2025).

Toussaint, C.M., Helou, A., Tucker, M.A. & Reeves, J.T. (2021) 'Altitude, acute mountain sickness, and acetazolamide: recommendations for rapid ascent', *High Altitude Medicine & Biology*, 22(1), pp. 5–13. https://doi.org/10.1089/ham.2019.0123.

Vidt, D.G. (1981) 'Mechanism of action, pharmacokinetics, adverse effects, and therapeutic uses of amiloride hydrochloride', *Pharmacotherapy*, 1(3), pp. 179–187. https://doi.org/10.1002/j.1875-9114.1981.tb02539.x.

Yue, C.S., Huynh, H.H., Raymond, C., Charbonneau, L. & Roy, L. (2013) 'Population pharmacokinetic and pharmacodynamic modeling of acetazolamide in peritoneal dialysis patients and healthy volunteers', *Journal of Pharmacy & Pharmaceutical Sciences*, 16(1), pp. 89–98. https://doi.org/10.18433/J3QG7Z.

Drugs Acting on Blood 9

9.1 Blood Products

9.1.1 Red Cell Concentrate

Also known as: Packed Red Cells (PRC)

Red cell concentrate is the most commonly transfused blood product and forms the cornerstone of red cell replacement therapy. It consists of concentrated erythrocytes suspended in additive solution with a small volume of plasma. RCC is primarily used to restore oxygen-carrying capacity in patients with acute blood loss or symptomatic anaemia. A single unit typically increases haemoglobin by approximately 1 g/dL (10 g/L) (Naidech et al. 2008).

Indications

RCC is indicated for acute haemorrhage (e.g. trauma, surgery, obstetric bleeding), symptomatic anaemia—particularly when haemoglobin levels fall below 8.0 g/dL—and in chronic anaemias such as myelodysplasia or haemoglobinopathies, where individualised thresholds apply. It may also be used preoperatively in patients with ischaemic heart disease or other high-risk conditions.

Volume, Storage, and Compatibility

Each unit contains approximately 330 mL and is stored at 2–6 °C in blood bank refrigerators for up to 35 days. Compatibility testing based on ABO and Rh blood group systems is essential. Crossmatching is required prior to transfusion unless emergency O-negative blood is used.

Modified Preparations

All RCC units are now leucodepleted to reduce febrile non-haemolytic transfusion reactions and CMV transmission. Additional modifications include irradiation, used to prevent transfusion-associated graft-versus-host disease (TA-GVHD) in specific

G. Browne, *PharmacologyPro*, https://doi.org/10.1007/978-3-032-10227-0_9

high-risk groups (e.g. stem cell transplant recipients, intrauterine transfusions, and patients with Hodgkin lymphoma) (Treleaven et al. 2011). CMV-negative products are indicated for neonates, transplant recipients, and certain pregnant women. Once irradiated, RCC must be transfused within 14 days.

Adverse Effects

Complications range from allergic and febrile reactions to serious events such as acute or delayed haemolytic transfusion reactions and transfusion-related acute lung injury (TRALI). Transfusion-associated circulatory overload (TACO) may occur, especially in older or frail patients. Metabolic effects include hyperkalaemia, hypocalcaemia due to citrate binding, and iron overload in patients requiring chronic transfusions. Infectious risks such as HIV and hepatitis are now extremely rare with modern screening. Graft-versus-host disease, although rare, is fatal in immunocompromised hosts and necessitates irradiated products.

Storage Lesions

Prolonged storage leads to changes in red cell properties, including a fall in pH, potassium leakage into the suspension fluid, and a decline in 2,3-DPG levels, which impairs oxygen release by shifting the haemoglobin dissociation curve to the left (van de Watering 2011). Membrane rigidity and reduced deformability can also impair microvascular perfusion.

Anaesthetic Considerations

Intraoperative transfusion decisions should be guided by haemodynamic status, surgical blood loss, and preoperative haemoglobin levels. Blood warmers are recommended for large-volume transfusions to prevent hypothermia. During massive transfusion, close monitoring of calcium and potassium is essential. Institutions should follow established massive transfusion protocols (MTPs). In patients at risk of bleeding, particularly those undergoing neuraxial anaesthesia, ensure cross-matched blood is available.

9.1.2 Fibrinogen

Fibrinogen is a soluble plasma glycoprotein synthesised in the liver and plays a central role in haemostasis. Upon activation by thrombin, fibrinogen is cleaved to form fibrin, which polymerises into a mesh that stabilises the blood clot. Beyond clot formation, fibrinogen also facilitates platelet aggregation by binding to the glycoprotein IIb/IIIa receptor on activated platelets. It is classified as an acute-phase reactant, with levels rising in response to inflammation, trauma, or pregnancy (Hofer et al. 2022).

Physiological Levels

Normal fibrinogen concentrations range from 2 to 4 g/L. In pregnancy, levels may physiologically rise to as high as 6 g/L (Hofer et al. 2022).

Indications for Replacement

Replacement of fibrinogen is indicated when levels fall below 1.5 g/L in the context of major bleeding. This is particularly relevant during trauma, postpartum haemorrhage, or disseminated intravascular coagulation (DIC). Early empirical replacement is also common in massive transfusion protocols (Leal-Noval et al. 2025).

Replacement Options

1. **Fibrinogen concentrate** is a lyophilised preparation reconstituted with sterile water and delivers a known quantity (typically 1 g per vial). It is virus-inactivated, rapidly available, and does not require blood group matching, making it increasingly preferred (Hensley et al. 2021).
2. **Cryoprecipitate** is derived from thawed plasma and contains fibrinogen along with Factor VIII and von Willebrand factor. However, its fibrinogen content is less predictable (~0.2–0.3 g per unit), and it requires thawing and ABO compatibility.
3. **Fresh frozen plasma (FFP)** also contains fibrinogen (~2 g/L), but large volumes are required to reach therapeutic fibrinogen levels, limiting its utility for targeted replacement.

Use in Massive Transfusion

In major haemorrhage protocols, fibrinogen is often administered early, with an empirical dose of 4 g (typically 4 vials of concentrate). Subsequent dosing can be guided by laboratory measurement using the Clauss assay or viscoelastic haemostatic tests such as ROTEM or TEG (Leal-Noval et al. 2025).

Administration Notes

Fibrinogen concentrate should be gently swirled, not shaken, during reconstitution. Once fully dissolved, it can be administered rapidly.

Adverse Effects

Side effects are rare but include allergic reactions such as fever, nausea, vomiting, or chills. Serious reactions may involve anaphylaxis or thromboembolic events, including deep vein thrombosis, pulmonary embolism, stroke, myocardial infarction, or peripheral arterial thrombosis (Hensley et al. 2021).

Summary

Fibrinogen plays an essential role in both clot formation and platelet aggregation. In bleeding patients, especially during massive transfusion, prompt fibrinogen replacement improves haemostatic efficacy. Fibrinogen concentrate is generally favoured due to its reliable dosing, ease of preparation, and favourable safety profile compared with cryoprecipitate or FFP (Hensley et al. 2021).

9.1.3 Platelets

Platelets are small anuclear cell fragments derived from megakaryocytes and play a central role in primary haemostasis. They adhere to damaged endothelium, aggregate, and recruit additional platelets to form a haemostatic plug. These actions are facilitated by interactions with von Willebrand factor and fibrinogen. Platelet transfusion is used to prevent or treat bleeding associated with thrombocytopenia or platelet dysfunction (Estcourt et al. 2017).

Indications for Transfusion

Prophylactic platelet transfusion is recommended when the platelet count falls below 10,000/uL to reduce the risk of spontaneous bleeding. In the setting of active bleeding, transfusion is typically indicated at platelet counts below 50,000/uL. Thresholds vary depending on procedural risk. For central venous catheter insertion, a count above 20,000/uL is usually sufficient. Major non-neurological surgery requires levels above 50,000/uL, while neurosurgical or ophthalmic procedures typically warrant transfusion if platelets are below 100,000/uL. For neuraxial anaesthesia, a count exceeding 80,000/uL is generally advised to minimise the risk of spinal haematoma (Estcourt et al. 2017).

Compatibility and Sourcing

ABO compatibility is preferred for platelet transfusion, though RhD matching is of lesser importance. In emergencies, unmatched platelets can be given. Platelets may be obtained either through pooling from multiple whole blood donations (pooled platelets) or via apheresis from a single donor (Schiffer et al. 2018).

Storage and Handling

Platelets are stored at 20–24 °C in specialised incubators and kept under continuous agitation to prevent clumping. Each unit typically has a volume of approximately 300 mL. A therapeutic dose often requires pooling from four donors. The standard shelf life is 5 days, though this may extend to 7 days if the product passes bacterial screening protocols. Because platelets are stored at room temperature, the risk of bacterial contamination is significantly higher compared with other blood products (Jacobs et al. 2011).

Anaesthetic Considerations

Platelet function and count are critical in perioperative management. Neuraxial anaesthesia carries a risk of spinal haematoma in thrombocytopenic patients, with a platelet threshold of 80,000/uL widely considered acceptable. Platelet dysfunction due to antiplatelet agents or uraemia may necessitate transfusion even in the presence of normal counts. In massive transfusion protocols, early administration of platelets is essential to maintain haemostasis and prevent dilutional coagulopathy (Estcourt et al. 2017).

Adverse Effects

Although generally well tolerated, platelet transfusion may cause complications. These include febrile non-haemolytic reactions, allergic reactions, anaphylaxis, transfusion-associated circulatory overload (TACO), transfusion-related acute lung injury (TRALI), and, more rarely, haemolytic reactions. The risk of sepsis due to bacterial contamination is higher with platelets than with other blood components due to storage at room temperature (Jacobs et al. 2011).

Summary

Platelet transfusions are a cornerstone of haemostatic therapy in both elective and emergency clinical settings. Appropriate threshold-based transfusion, consideration of function over count in certain scenarios, and close attention to compatibility, storage, and potential adverse effects are all critical to safe and effective use (Schiffer et al. 2018).

9.1.4 Fresh Frozen Plasma

Fresh Frozen Plasma (FFP) is the acellular, protein-rich component of human blood obtained by centrifugation and frozen within 8 h of collection. It contains all coagulation factors, including fibrinogen, prothrombin, factors V, VII, VIII, IX, X, XI, XII, and XIII, as well as albumin, immunoglobulins, and other plasma proteins (O'Shaughnessy et al. 2004). FFP can be derived from whole blood or collected by apheresis and must be ABO-compatible to reduce the risk of haemolytic reactions.

Storage and Handling

FFP is stored at or below −25 °C to preserve clotting factor activity and remains viable for up to 36 months in its frozen state. Once thawed, it should be kept at 1–6 °C and used within 24 h. Each unit typically contains approximately 275 mL. Prior to transfusion, standard blood group compatibility testing is required. Administration should follow transfusion protocols, including the use of appropriate filters to prevent the infusion of microaggregates or clots (Hunt et al. 2015).

Indications for Use

FFP is indicated in the management of active bleeding with documented coagulopathy, as part of massive transfusion protocols (MTP), or in disseminated intravascular coagulation (DIC). It is also used in patients with liver disease where clotting factor production is impaired, and in congenital or acquired deficiencies of multiple clotting factors—particularly when specific factor concentrates are unavailable. In thrombotic thrombocytopenic purpura (TTP), FFP is used in plasma exchange therapy. It may also be used to reverse warfarin anticoagulation in emergency settings if prothrombin complex concentrate (PCC) is not accessible (Hofer et al. 2021).

Dosing and Monitoring
A typical dose is 15 mL/kg, which equates to around 4 units for an average adult. Larger volumes may be needed in cases of massive haemorrhage. The efficacy of FFP can be monitored using standard coagulation assays such as prothrombin time (PT), activated partial thromboplastin time (aPTT), or specific factor levels if available (Hunt et al. 2015).

Contraindications and Cautions
FFP should not be used as a simple plasma expander or for nutritional support. It is not appropriate for isolated clotting factor deficiencies when dedicated concentrates exist. Likewise, it is not recommended for routine reversal of warfarin in the absence of bleeding or prior to minor procedures, particularly when PCC is available (O'Shaughnessy et al. 2004).

Adverse Effects
Complications include allergic reactions such as urticaria, flushing, and fever. Anaphylaxis is rare but potentially life-threatening. FFP is associated with transfusion-related acute lung injury (TRALI), a leading cause of transfusion-associated mortality, and transfusion-associated circulatory overload (TACO), especially in elderly or cardiac patients. Other risks include febrile non-haemolytic transfusion reactions, haemolysis from ABO incompatibility, and sepsis due to bacterial contamination (although rare with proper screening) (Hofer et al. 2021). In rare instances, FFP may also contribute to hyperfibrinolysis or thrombosis.

Summary
Fresh Frozen Plasma is an essential blood product for correcting complex coagulation abnormalities, particularly in critical care, trauma, and perioperative settings. Its use should be based on clinical and laboratory evidence of coagulopathy and guided by robust transfusion protocols to optimise safety and efficacy (O'Shaughnessy et al. 2004; Hofer et al. 2021; Hunt et al. 2015).

9.1.5 Prothrombin Complex Concentrate

Also known as 4-factor PCC and available under brand names such as Octaplex and Beriplex, Prothrombin Complex Concentrate is a lyophilised plasma-derived product containing four essential vitamin K–dependent clotting factors—Factors II, VII, IX, and X—as well as the natural anticoagulants protein C and protein S (Samama 2008). It is primarily indicated for the rapid reversal of warfarin and other vitamin K antagonists and is increasingly used in acute bleeding scenarios where rapid haemostatic correction is required.

Indications
PCC is indicated for the emergency reversal of warfarin anticoagulation in patients requiring urgent surgery or those presenting with life-threatening bleeding such as

intracranial haemorrhage (Keeling et al. 2011). It may also be used off-label in the setting of liver disease–related coagulopathy or as part of a massive transfusion protocol (MTP), particularly when the INR is elevated and fresh frozen plasma (FFP) is unavailable or contraindicated.

Mechanism of Action
PCC works by replenishing deficient vitamin K–dependent clotting factors, thereby restoring thrombin generation and improving haemostatic function. It provides rapid correction of prothrombin time (PT) and international normalized ratio (INR), especially when combined with intravenous vitamin K (typically 10 mg IV), which is necessary for sustained reversal (Samama 2008).

Pharmacokinetics
PCC is administered intravenously and has a rapid onset of action—typically within 15–30 min. Its duration depends on the patient's underlying coagulation status and the concurrent use of vitamin K. The clotting factors are metabolised in the liver through natural degradation pathways.

Dosing
Dosing is weight- and INR-dependent. Common regimens include 25 IU/kg for INR 2–4, 35 IU/kg for INR 4–6, and 50 IU/kg for INR >6. A maximum dose of 3000 IU is typically observed to mitigate thrombotic risk. INR should be reassessed 30–60 min post-infusion to confirm efficacy (Sarode et al. 2013).

Advantages Over FFP
PCC offers several practical and clinical advantages compared to FFP: it requires a smaller volume for administration (reducing the risk of transfusion-associated circulatory overload), acts more rapidly, and does not require blood group matching. It is also virus-inactivated and easier to store and reconstitute, with fewer associated transfusion-related complications (Samama 2008; Sarode et al. 2013).

Adverse Effects
Although generally well tolerated, PCC carries a risk of thromboembolic complications including deep vein thrombosis (DVT), pulmonary embolism, myocardial infarction, and stroke. Rare adverse events include hypersensitivity reactions (such as anaphylaxis) and disseminated intravascular coagulation (DIC), particularly if used inappropriately or in excessive doses (Sarode et al. 2013).

Storage and Preparation
PCC is supplied as a lyophilised powder in glass vials (typically 500 IU or 1000 IU) and should be reconstituted with sterile water—usually 20–40 mL provided in the kit. The solution should be used within 3 h of reconstitution. Vials are stored refrigerated and have a long shelf life of up to 2–3 years (Samama 2008).

Anaesthetic Considerations

In the perioperative setting, PCC is particularly useful in anticoagulated patients requiring urgent or emergency surgery (e.g. hip fracture in a patient on warfarin). Its rapid onset facilitates timely reversal, but care must be taken in patients with mechanical heart valves or a history of thromboembolic events. Co-administration of vitamin K is essential to sustain haemostatic correction and prevent rebound anticoagulation. INR monitoring before and after administration ensures safe and effective dosing (Keeling et al. 2011).

9.1.6 Tranexamic Acid (TXA)

Tranexamic acid is a synthetic lysine analogue that acts as a potent antifibrinolytic agent. It stabilises blood clots by inhibiting fibrinolysis and is widely used across surgical, trauma, and obstetric settings to reduce bleeding and minimise transfusion requirements (CRASH-2 Trial Collaborators 2010; WOMAN Trial Collaborators 2017).

Mechanism of Action

Tranexamic acid works by reversibly binding to lysine-binding sites on plasminogen, thereby blocking its conversion to plasmin—the enzyme responsible for degrading fibrin clots. By inhibiting plasmin-mediated fibrinolysis, it helps preserve clot integrity and reduce blood loss (Roberts 2015).

Uses and Indications

Tranexamic acid is indicated in a variety of bleeding contexts. It is a key intervention in major trauma with haemorrhage, ideally administered within 3 h of injury (CRASH-2 Trial Collaborators 2010). It is routinely used to reduce perioperative blood loss in orthopaedic, cardiac, and gynaecological surgery, and in the management of postpartum haemorrhage (WOMAN Trial Collaborators 2017). Other indications include heavy menstrual bleeding, epistaxis, dental procedures in patients with bleeding disorders, and as adjunct therapy in inherited coagulopathies such as von Willebrand disease and mild haemophilia. It may also be used during liver surgery or transplantation to minimise fibrinolytic bleeding (Roberts 2015).

Pharmacokinetics

Tranexamic acid is available in intravenous, oral, and topical formulations. Oral bioavailability ranges from 30% to 50%. It has a plasma half-life of approximately 2–3 h and is eliminated unchanged via renal excretion. Dose adjustments are necessary in patients with impaired renal function.

Dosing

For trauma or perioperative bleeding, the standard regimen is 1 g IV over 10 min followed by a continuous infusion of 1 g over 8 h (CRASH-2 Trial Collaborators

2010). In postpartum haemorrhage, 1 g IV is administered at the onset of bleeding, with a second 1 g dose given if bleeding persists after 30 min or recurs within 24 h (WOMAN Trial Collaborators 2017). For non-surgical indications such as menorrhagia, oral doses typically range from 500 mg to 1 g taken two to three times daily for 3–5 days.

Adverse Effects
Common side effects include gastrointestinal upset (nausea, vomiting, diarrhoea) and, rarely, visual disturbances such as colour vision changes. Seizures have been reported in high-dose settings, particularly during cardiac surgery. Although the overall risk of thrombosis is low, caution is advised in patients with a history of thromboembolic disease or those receiving oestrogen-containing contraceptives (Roberts 2015).

Contraindications and Cautions
Tranexamic acid is contraindicated in patients with active thromboembolic disease (e.g. DVT, pulmonary embolism, stroke), severe renal impairment, or a history of seizures. Caution is warranted in patients at increased risk of thrombosis, particularly when used in combination with hormonal therapies.

Anaesthetic Considerations
Tranexamic acid is a cornerstone of blood conservation strategies in modern anaesthesia. Its perioperative use has been shown to reduce blood loss and the need for transfusion in high-risk procedures (CRASH-2 Trial Collaborators 2010; WOMAN Trial Collaborators 2017). Anaesthetists should monitor renal function for dose adjustment and remain vigilant for rare adverse effects such as seizures or visual disturbances during prolonged or high-dose infusions.

Summary
With a favourable safety profile, low cost, and proven efficacy in reducing perioperative and trauma-related bleeding, tranexamic acid has become an indispensable tool in anaesthetic, surgical, and critical care practice. Its timely administration can improve outcomes and reduce transfusion-related morbidity (Roberts 2015; CRASH-2 Trial Collaborators 2010; WOMAN Trial Collaborators 2017).

9.2 Anticoagulant Drugs

Anticoagulants are a class of medications that interfere with the coagulation cascade, thereby reducing the formation of fibrin clots and prolonging clotting time. They are essential in both prophylactic and therapeutic settings to manage and prevent thromboembolic disorders. Their clinical utility spans cardiology, haematology, nephrology, anaesthesia, and critical care (Chen et al. 2020).

Clinical Indications
Common indications for anticoagulation include atrial fibrillation (to reduce the risk of cardioembolic stroke), deep vein thrombosis (DVT), and pulmonary embolism (PE). They are also used in patients with hypercoagulable states such as Factor V Leiden mutation or antiphospholipid syndrome, and in those with coronary artery disease, often alongside antiplatelet agents. Anticoagulants play a critical role in maintaining patency of vascular and extracorporeal circuits during haemodialysis, cardiopulmonary bypass (CPB), and extracorporeal membrane oxygenation (ECMO). Additionally, they are essential in preventing thrombosis following the insertion of coronary or peripheral vascular stents (Chen et al. 2020).

Anaesthetic Considerations
In anaesthetic practice, anticoagulants pose significant implications for procedural safety. Neuraxial anaesthesia (spinal and epidural techniques) requires meticulous timing relative to the last anticoagulant dose due to the risk of spinal haematoma. Perioperative management often necessitates temporary cessation of anticoagulation, with or without bridging therapy, depending on the agent used and the patient's thromboembolic risk (Kim 2020). Reversal strategies must be readily available in the event of bleeding or the need for urgent surgery; some anticoagulants have specific reversal agents (e.g. idarucizumab for dabigatran, andexanet alfa for factor Xa inhibitors) (Levy et al. 2018). Monitoring requirements vary—warfarin necessitates regular INR checks, heparin requires aPTT or anti-Xa monitoring, while direct oral anticoagulants (DOACs) generally do not require routine laboratory monitoring (Kim 2020) (Table 9.1).

9.2.1 Factor Xa Inhibitors

Factor Xa inhibitors are a class of Direct Oral Anticoagulants (DOACs) that act by selectively and reversibly inhibiting Factor Xa—a pivotal enzyme in the coagulation cascade. By preventing the conversion of prothrombin to thrombin, these agents reduce thrombin generation and fibrin clot formation. They also impair thrombin-mediated platelet activation. The class includes rivaroxaban, apixaban, and edoxaban; this section focuses primarily on rivaroxaban (Mueck et al. 2014).

Table 9.1 Classes of anticoagulants

Class	Examples	Mechanism
Traditional Anticoagulants	Heparin, LMWH, Warfarin	Potentiation of antithrombin III (Heparin), Vitamin K inhibition (Warfarin)
Direct Oral Anticoagulants (DOACs)	Apixaban, Rivaroxaban, Edoxaban, Dabigatran	Direct Xa or thrombin inhibition
Synthetic Factor Xa Inhibitor	Fondaparinux	Selective inhibition of factor Xa

Clinical Uses

Factor Xa inhibitors are widely used in the treatment and secondary prevention of venous thromboembolism (VTE), including deep vein thrombosis (DVT) and pulmonary embolism (PE). They are also indicated for stroke prevention in patients with non-valvular atrial fibrillation, and for thromboprophylaxis following major orthopaedic procedures such as hip or knee replacement. Additionally, rivaroxaban is approved for reducing the risk of major cardiovascular events in patients with chronic coronary or peripheral artery disease (Patel et al. 2011).

Pharmacokinetics

Rivaroxaban has high oral bioavailability (~90%), especially when taken with food. Peak plasma concentrations are achieved within 2–4 h. It is extensively protein-bound (~95%) and undergoes hepatic metabolism via CYP3A4, CYP2J2, and non-CYP pathways. Approximately one-third of the dose is excreted unchanged in the urine, with the remainder metabolised and eliminated via both renal and hepatobiliary routes. The elimination half-life is 7–11 h, which may be prolonged in elderly patients or those with renal impairment (Mueck et al. 2014).

Adverse Effects

Bleeding is the most significant adverse effect and may involve gastrointestinal, intracranial, or other sites. Hepatotoxicity, including elevated transaminases, has been reported. Gastrointestinal symptoms such as nausea, vomiting, and abdominal discomfort are relatively common. Rare but serious haematological effects include agranulocytosis and thrombocytopenia. Hypersensitivity reactions (including anaphylaxis and angioedema) and severe dermatological events such as Stevens–Johnson syndrome and DRESS syndrome have also been described (Patel et al. 2011).

Anaesthetic Considerations

In the perioperative setting, particular caution is required. Neuraxial anaesthesia is contraindicated unless sufficient time has elapsed since the last dose—typically at least 72 h, especially in patients with renal impairment. For emergency surgery or procedures with high bleeding risk, elective delays are preferred. Where reversal is needed, specific agents include andexanet alfa, a recombinant Factor Xa decoy protein approved for apixaban and rivaroxaban, though it carries a black box warning for thromboembolic complications. Prothrombin Complex Concentrate (PCC) may be used off-label in life-threatening bleeding. Routine coagulation monitoring is not required, but anti-Xa levels or prothrombin time (PT) may offer insight into anticoagulant activity in urgent clinical contexts (Kozek-Langenecker et al. 2017) (Tables 9.2 and 9.3).

Table 9.2 Doses of FXa inhibitors

Drug	Typical dose	Prophylaxis dose
Rivaroxaban	20 mg once daily (treatment)	10 mg once daily (e.g. post-op)
Apixaban	5–10 mg twice daily	2.5 mg twice daily
Edoxaban	60 mg once daily	Not routinely used for prophylaxis

Table 9.3 Characteristics of FXa inhibitors

Feature	Rivaroxaban	Apixaban	Edoxaban
Drug Class	Direct Factor Xa Inhibitor	Direct Factor Xa Inhibitor	Direct Factor Xa Inhibitor
Trade Name	Xarelto	Eliquis	Lixiana (EU) / Savaysa (US)
Indications	AF (non-valvular) DVT/PE treatment & prophylaxis Post-op thromboprophylaxis	AF (non-valvular) DVT/PE treatment & prophylaxis Post-op thromboprophylaxis	AF (non-valvular) DVT/PE treatment & prophylaxis
Typical Dose	20 mg OD with food (AF, DVT/PE) 10 mg OD (post-op prophylaxis)	5 mg BD (standard) 2.5 mg BD (dose reduction criteria)	60 mg OD 30 mg OD (renal impairment or <60 kg)
Oral Bioavailability	~90% (improved with food)	~50%	~62%
Dosing Frequency	Once daily	Twice daily	Once daily
Renal Elimination	~33%	~27%	~50%
Hepatic Metabolism	CYP3A4 + P-gp	CYP3A4 + P-gp	Minimal CYP3A4
Half-Life	7–11 h	9–14 h	10–14 h
Reversal Agent	Andexanet alfa PCC (off-label)	Andexanet alfa PCC (off-label)	No specific reversal PCC (off-label)
Neuraxial Anaesthesia	Hold ≥72 h pre−/post-block	Hold ≥72 h pre−/post-block	Hold ≥72 h pre−/post-block
Major Side Effects	Bleeding, ↑LFTs, SJS, GI upset	Bleeding, rash, GI upset, SJS	Bleeding, GI upset
Use in Renal Impairment	Dose adjust or avoid if CrCl <30 ml/min	Safer in renal impairment	Dose reduce if CrCl 15–50 ml/min
Pregnancy/ Breastfeeding	Contraindicated	Contraindicated	Contraindicated
Monitoring	Not routinely required	Not routinely required	Not routinely required

9.2.2 Direct Thrombin Inhibitors

Example: Dabigatran (Pradaxa)

Direct thrombin inhibitors represent a class of oral anticoagulants that directly block thrombin (Factor IIa), a central enzyme in the coagulation cascade. Dabigatran is the most clinically used agent in this category. Unlike heparin, which requires antithrombin as a cofactor, dabigatran binds directly to thrombin, inhibiting the conversion of fibrinogen to fibrin and also suppressing thrombin-induced platelet aggregation (Stangier et al. 2007).

Clinical Uses

Dabigatran is indicated for the prevention of stroke and systemic embolism in patients with non-valvular atrial fibrillation. It is also approved for the treatment and secondary prevention of deep vein thrombosis (DVT) and pulmonary embolism (PE). It is not recommended in patients with mechanical heart valves due to increased risk of thromboembolic and bleeding complications (Connolly et al. 2009).

Pharmacokinetics

Dabigatran is administered orally as a prodrug (dabigatran etexilate) and has a low oral bioavailability (<10%). Peak plasma concentrations are typically reached within 2–3 h. The drug is predominantly cleared via the kidneys (approximately 80%), with an elimination half-life of around 15 h, which may be prolonged in renal impairment. Dose adjustment is necessary in patients with reduced renal function (Stangier et al. 2007).

Adverse Effects

Gastrointestinal symptoms such as dyspepsia, nausea, and vomiting are relatively common. The most significant adverse effect is bleeding, particularly from the gastrointestinal tract. Dabigatran is contraindicated in patients with severe renal impairment (eGFR <30 mL/min/1.73 m^2). Hypersensitivity reactions including rash and anaphylaxis are rare (Connolly et al. 2009).

Reversal and Monitoring

Routine coagulation monitoring is not required due to the drug's predictable pharmacokinetics. However, in emergencies, activated partial thromboplastin time (aPTT) may offer a rough estimate of anticoagulant activity. Idarucizumab (Praxbind) is a specific monoclonal antibody fragment that provides immediate reversal of dabigatran's anticoagulant effect and is used in cases of life-threatening bleeding or urgent surgery (Pollack et al. 2015).

Dosing

The standard dose is 150 mg orally twice daily. In patients with moderate renal impairment or aged ≥75 years, a reduced dose of 110 mg twice daily is typically used (Stangier et al. 2007).

Anaesthetic Considerations

In patients undergoing neuraxial anaesthesia, dabigatran should be discontinued at least 72 h in advance if renal function is normal. In those with renal impairment, a longer interval is recommended. Residual anticoagulant activity must be excluded before performing spinal or epidural procedures. Neuraxial blockade is contraindicated in patients with ongoing dabigatran effect due to the risk of spinal haematoma (Kozek-Langenecker et al. 2017—already cited in Sect. 9.2.1).

9.2.3 Heparin

Heparin is a naturally occurring glycosaminoglycan that exerts anticoagulant effects by potentiating antithrombin III (ATIII), which in turn inhibits thrombin (Factor IIa) and Factor Xa. It is available in two clinically distinct forms: unfractionated heparin (UFH) and low-molecular-weight heparin (LMWH), each with different pharmacokinetic profiles and monitoring requirements (Hirsh and Raschke 2004).

Forms

Unfractionated Heparin (UFH) is a large, heterogeneous molecule (~15,000 Da) administered intravenously. It has a short and variable half-life and requires close monitoring using activated partial thromboplastin time (aPTT) or activated clotting time (ACT) (Kitchen et al. 1999).

Low-Molecular-Weight Heparin (LMWH) includes preparations such as enoxaparin, tinzaparin, and dalteparin. These smaller fragments (3000–8000 Da) are administered subcutaneously, exhibit more predictable pharmacokinetics, and do not require routine monitoring (Weitz 1997).

Indications

Heparin is widely used for:

- VTE prophylaxis and treatment (including DVT and PE)
- Anticoagulation in acute coronary syndromes and atrial fibrillation
- Bridging therapy during interruption of long-term anticoagulation (e.g. perioperative warfarin management)
- Priming of extracorporeal circuits, including dialysis, ECMO, and cardiopulmonary bypass (Hirsh and Raschke 2004).

Mechanism of Action

Heparin binds to antithrombin III, inducing a conformational change that accelerates its inhibition of coagulation enzymes. UFH inhibits both Factor IIa (thrombin) and Factor Xa effectively, whereas LMWH has greater selectivity for Factor Xa (Hirsh and Raschke 2004).

Table 9.4 Pharmacokinetics of Heparin

Property	UFH	LMWH
Route	IV only	SC (main), IV
Onset	Immediate (IV)	~1–2
Half-life	30–90 min	4–6 h
Monitoring	aPTT / ACT	None (unless renal impairment, pregnancy, or obesity)
Clearance	Hepatic, renal	Primarily renal

Pharmacokinetics

UFH is administered intravenously and has a rapid onset but requires frequent dose adjustments due to variable binding to plasma proteins and endothelium. LMWH, given subcutaneously, offers better bioavailability, a longer half-life, and more predictable effects (Weitz 1997) (Table 9.4).

Side Effects

Bleeding is the most common adverse effect. Heparin-induced thrombocytopenia (HIT) is a serious immune-mediated complication, typically occurring 4–10 days after initiation (Warkentin and Greinacher 2004). Other adverse effects include osteoporosis with prolonged use, hyperkalaemia, elevated liver transaminases, and local injection site reactions (Warkentin and Greinacher 2004).

Anaesthetic Considerations

Neuraxial anaesthesia poses a risk of spinal haematoma in anticoagulated patients. For UFH, a minimum of 4–6 h should elapse before spinal or epidural placement. For LMWH, the interval depends on dose: 12 h for prophylactic and 24 h for therapeutic regimens. Catheters should not be removed until the same intervals have passed. The risk increases if neuraxial techniques are combined with anticoagulation (Horlocker et al. 2018).

Reversal

Protamine sulphate is the primary reversal agent. It fully neutralises recent UFH (1 mg protamine per 100 units heparin given within the past 4 h) and partially reverses LMWH (approximately 60%). Care must be taken to avoid hypotension and allergic reactions during administration (Hirsh and Raschke 2004).

Dosing

Unfractionated Heparin (UFH):

- Treatment: Initial IV bolus (e.g. 5000 units), followed by continuous infusion, adjusted to maintain aPTT 1.5–2.5× baseline (Hirsh and Raschke 2004).

Low-Molecular-Weight Heparin (LMWH):

- Prophylaxis (e.g. Enoxaparin): 40 mg SC once daily
- Treatment: Enoxaparin 1 mg/kg SC every 12 h; Tinzaparin 175 units/kg SC once daily (Hirsh and Raschke 2004).

9.2.4 Warfarin

Warfarin is a vitamin K antagonist that has long served as a cornerstone of oral anticoagulation therapy. Although largely supplanted by direct oral anticoagulants (DOACs) for many indications, warfarin remains the treatment of choice in specific clinical scenarios, particularly in patients with mechanical heart valves or antiphospholipid syndrome (Ageno et al. 2012).

Uses

Warfarin is used for both treatment and secondary prevention of venous and arterial thromboembolic conditions. Indications include atrial fibrillation (particularly in the presence of valvular disease), deep vein thrombosis (DVT), pulmonary embolism (PE), and the prevention of thromboembolism in patients with mechanical heart valves. It also plays a role in managing antiphospholipid syndrome and may be used for secondary prevention following myocardial infarction or ischaemic stroke (Ageno et al. 2012).

Mechanism of Action

Warfarin inhibits the enzyme Vitamin K Epoxide Reductase Complex 1 (VKORC1), which blocks the regeneration of reduced vitamin K. This prevents the γ-carboxylation of vitamin K–dependent clotting factors—specifically factors II, VII, IX, and X—as well as the natural anticoagulants Protein C and Protein S. Early in therapy, Protein C and S levels decline faster than procoagulant factors, transiently increasing thrombotic risk and necessitating bridging anticoagulation with heparin in high-risk patients (Johnson et al. 2011).

Pharmacokinetics

Administered orally with high bioavailability (~90%), warfarin is extensively protein-bound (~99%) and undergoes hepatic metabolism primarily via CYP2C9, with contributions from CYP1A2 and CYP3A4. Its anticoagulant effect has a long functional half-life of approximately 60 h, though terminal elimination may extend up to one week. Inactive metabolites are excreted renally (Johnson et al. 2011).

Side Effects

The primary risk is haemorrhage, which is dose-dependent and may be life-threatening. Other notable adverse effects include warfarin-induced skin necrosis, purple toe syndrome, osteoporosis with long-term use, and teratogenicity (contraindicated in pregnancy, especially during the first trimester) (Patel et al. 2017).

Interactions and Considerations

Warfarin is highly susceptible to drug and dietary interactions. CYP450 inducers (e.g., rifampicin, carbamazepine) reduce its effect, while inhibitors (e.g., amiodarone, macrolides) enhance it. Displacement from plasma proteins by other drugs such as NSAIDs increases free warfarin levels. Dietary vitamin K—particularly

Table 9.5 INR Targets with Warfarin

Indication	Target INR (Range)
Atrial Fibrillation, DVT, PE, Bioprosthetic valves	2.5 (range: 2.0–3.0)
Mechanical (metallic) valves, Ball-and-cage valves	3.0 (range: 2.5–3.5)

from green leafy vegetables—can antagonise its effects. Originally developed as a rodenticide, warfarin requires meticulous monitoring to ensure efficacy and safety (Ageno et al. 2012; Johnson et al. 2011).

Reversal Agents

- Vitamin K (phytomenadione)—administered orally or intravenously
- Prothrombin Complex Concentrate (PCC)—preferred for rapid reversal in bleeding
- Fresh Frozen Plasma (FFP)—alternative when PCC is unavailable
- Frequent INR monitoring is essential to guide therapy and assess reversal effectiveness (Ageno et al. 2012).

Anaesthesia Considerations
Warfarin must be discontinued at least 5 days before elective surgery, with the INR <1.4 required for safe neuraxial anaesthesia. In patients at high thrombotic risk, LMWH bridging may be indicated. Resumption postoperatively requires individualised risk–benefit analysis, balancing bleeding risk with thromboembolic protection (Horlocker et al. 2018—already cited in Heparin section).

Dosing
Dosing is highly individualised, generally ranging from 2 to 10 mg once daily, adjusted based on INR targets (typically 2.0–3.0). Frequent monitoring is essential due to variability in metabolism and numerous interactions (Johnson et al. 2011) (Table 9.5).

9.3 Antiplatelet Drugs

Antiplatelet agents are fundamental in the prevention and treatment of arterial thromboembolic events. They are particularly effective in conditions where platelet activation and aggregation play a central pathogenic role, such as myocardial infarction, ischaemic stroke, and peripheral arterial disease (Antithrombotic Trialists' Collaboration 2002). In contrast to anticoagulants, which inhibit the coagulation cascade and are more effective in preventing venous thromboembolism, antiplatelets primarily inhibit platelet plug formation, making them more effective for arterial thrombosis.

Indications

Antiplatelet therapy is commonly employed in a range of cardiovascular and cerebrovascular conditions, including:

- Myocardial ischaemia, such as angina and acute coronary syndromes (ACS)
- Secondary prevention following myocardial infarction or ischaemic stroke
- Percutaneous coronary intervention (PCI) and coronary stenting
- Transient ischaemic attacks (TIA)
- Peripheral vascular disease
- Postoperative management after coronary artery bypass grafting (CABG) or valve surgery
- Selected cases of pulmonary embolism, especially those involving atrial fibrillation or vascular stents
- Patients supported by mechanical circulatory devices, such as intra-aortic balloon pumps or left ventricular assist devices (LVADs) (Levine et al. 2016; Antithrombotic Trialists' Collaboration 2002).

Mechanism of Action

Antiplatelet drugs inhibit one or more stages of platelet activation, adhesion, or aggregation, thereby reducing the formation of platelet-rich thrombi. They exert their effects via diverse pathways, such as:

- Cyclooxygenase (COX-1) inhibition (e.g. aspirin) (Patrono and Baigent 2019)
- P2Y12 receptor blockade (e.g. clopidogrel, ticagrelor) (Levine et al. 2016)
- Glycoprotein IIb/IIIa inhibition
- Thromboxane receptor antagonism (Patrono and Baigent 2019) (Table 9.6)

Dual Antiplatelet Therapy (DAPT)

DAPT refers to the combination of aspirin and a P2Y12 receptor inhibitor (such as clopidogrel, prasugrel, or ticagrelor). It is employed in high-risk scenarios to enhance antiplatelet efficacy, particularly in:

Table 9.6 Classes of antiplatelet agents

Class	Example Drugs	Mechanism
COX Inhibitors	Aspirin	Irreversibly inhibits COX-1 → ↓ thromboxane A2 → ↓ platelet activation
ADP Receptor (P2Y12) Inhibitors	Clopidogrel, Prasugrel, Ticagrelor	Block ADP binding to P2Y12 → inhibits GPIIb/IIIa activation and aggregation
GPIIb/IIIa Inhibitors	Abciximab, Tirofiban	Block fibrinogen and vWF binding to GPIIb/IIIa → inhibit final common pathway
PDE Inhibitors	Dipyridamole, Cilostazol	↑ cAMP → ↓ platelet activation and vasodilation

- Acute coronary syndrome (ACS)
- Recent coronary stenting
- Secondary prevention post-MI or stroke

Duration of DAPT is guided by the underlying indication, stent type, and individual bleeding risk (Valgimigli et al. 2018).

Anaesthetic and Perioperative Considerations
Management of antiplatelet therapy in the perioperative and anaesthetic context requires careful individualisation.

- Aspirin monotherapy is generally considered safe for neuraxial anaesthesia and does not necessitate discontinuation in most cases (Albaladejo et al. 2011).
- P2Y12 inhibitors such as clopidogrel, ticagrelor, or prasugrel should typically be withheld for 5–7 days prior to neuraxial block to reduce the risk of spinal haematoma (Kietaibl et al. 2022).
- Bridging therapy may be considered in high thrombotic risk patients undergoing major surgery (Albaladejo et al. 2011).

Patients with renal impairment, hepatic dysfunction, or haematological malignancies may exhibit altered platelet function and enhanced bleeding risk, warranting closer monitoring (Kietaibl et al. 2022).

9.3.1 COX Inhibitors

The principal antiplatelet agent in this class is aspirin (acetylsalicylic acid). It is widely employed for both primary and secondary prevention of arterial thrombotic events, including myocardial infarction (MI) and ischaemic stroke, due to its potent and irreversible inhibition of platelet function (Antithrombotic Trialists' Collaboration 2002). Indications include acute coronary syndromes (with or without PCI), secondary prevention after TIA or stroke, peripheral arterial disease, and thromboprophylaxis in atrial fibrillation where anticoagulants are contraindicated. At higher doses, aspirin also exerts anti-inflammatory and analgesic effects, although this is not its primary use in modern cardiovascular medicine (Patrono and Baigent 2014).

Mechanism of Action
Aspirin acts by irreversibly inhibiting the cyclooxygenase-1 (COX-1) enzyme in platelets through acetylation of a serine residue. This blocks the synthesis of thromboxane A_2 (TXA_2), a potent vasoconstrictor and promoter of platelet aggregation. As platelets lack nuclei, they are unable to resynthesise COX-1, meaning aspirin's antiplatelet effect persists for the entire lifespan of the platelet (7–10 days) (Patrono and Baigent 2014). At higher concentrations, aspirin also inhibits COX-2, contributing to its anti-inflammatory and analgesic effects, though this is associated with greater gastrointestinal and renal toxicity.

Pharmacokinetics

Aspirin is typically administered orally, but rectal and intravenous formulations exist for selected clinical scenarios. It is rapidly absorbed from the stomach and small intestine, with a bioavailability of approximately 50–75% due to first-pass metabolism. Aspirin is ~90% protein bound and metabolised in the liver to salicyluric acid, which is then renally excreted. The parent compound has a short half-life of 15–20 min, whereas its active metabolite, salicylate, has a longer half-life (3–6 h), which may become prolonged at higher doses due to non-linear, saturable kinetics (Patrono and Baigent 2014).

Adverse Effects

The primary risk associated with aspirin is bleeding, particularly gastrointestinal and (less commonly) intracranial haemorrhage. Aspirin can cause gastritis, ulceration, and dyspepsia, and these effects are potentiated by concomitant NSAID or corticosteroid use. Renal function may be impaired, particularly in volume-depleted or elderly patients. Tinnitus and hearing disturbances (salicylism) can occur at higher doses. Hypersensitivity reactions, including asthma exacerbation and rash, are possible. A rare but serious complication is Reye's syndrome, which precludes its use in children under 16 years with viral illness (Antithrombotic Trialists' Collaboration 2002).

Anaesthetic Considerations

Due to its irreversible platelet inhibition, aspirin must be withheld for 5–7 days prior to neuraxial anaesthesia or surgeries with a high bleeding risk, unless ongoing therapy is critical (e.g., recent coronary stenting). For low-risk procedures, aspirin may be safely continued following local protocol. Patients on dual antiplatelet therapy (DAPT) with a P2Y12 inhibitor require multidisciplinary planning to determine whether and when to interrupt therapy preoperatively (Burger et al. 2005).

Contraindications

Absolute contraindications include active bleeding, peptic ulcer disease, severe renal or hepatic dysfunction, and known hypersensitivity to aspirin or NSAIDs. Use is also contraindicated in children under 16 years due to the risk of Reye's syndrome (Patrono and Baigent 2014) (Table 9.7).

Table 9.7 Doses of COX Inhibitors

Indication	Dose
Antiplatelet effect (ACS, stroke)	75–100 mg once daily
Acute MI	300 mg loading dose orally
Anti-inflammatory	300–600 mg every 4–6 h
Pain/fever	300–900 mg every 4–6 h

Note: Only low-dose aspirin (75–100 mg) is used for antiplatelet therapy

9.3.2 ADP Receptor Blockers

Drugs in this class include clopidogrel, prasugrel, and ticagrelor. These agents inhibit platelet aggregation and are widely used in cardiovascular disease. Their most common application is in dual antiplatelet therapy (DAPT), where they are combined with aspirin, particularly in patients with acute coronary syndromes (ACS) or following percutaneous coronary intervention (PCI) (Wallentin et al. 2009; Wiviott et al. 2007).

Uses

ADP receptor blockers are used to reduce thrombotic risk in acute coronary syndromes (STEMI, NSTEMI, and unstable angina), following coronary stenting, and in secondary prevention after myocardial infarction or stroke. They are also prescribed in peripheral arterial disease and in patients with a high atherothrombotic burden (Wiviott et al. 2007; Schüpke et al. 2019).

Mechanism of Action

These agents inhibit the $P2Y_{12}$ subtype of the ADP receptor on the platelet surface. This prevents ADP-mediated activation of the glycoprotein IIb/IIIa complex, thereby reducing platelet aggregation. Clopidogrel and prasugrel are irreversible prodrugs requiring metabolic activation, while ticagrelor is a reversible, direct-acting $P2Y_{12}$ antagonist with a faster onset and offset of action (Wallentin et al. 2009; Schüpke et al. 2019) (Table 9.8).

Side Effects

The principal adverse effect of $P2Y_{12}$ inhibitors is bleeding, including gastrointestinal and intracranial haemorrhage. Ticagrelor is also associated with dyspnoea, likely adenosine-mediated, and can cause bradyarrhythmias (Storey et al. 2010). Other effects may include rash, nausea, and rare cases of thrombocytopenia.

Table 9.8 Pharmacokinetics of ADP Receptor Blockers

Property	Ticagrelor	Clopidogrel	Prasugrel
Administration	Oral	Oral	Oral
Bioavailability	~35%	~50%	~80%
Onset of action	1–3 h	2–6 h	30 min – 1 h
Protein binding	>99%	~98%	~98%
Metabolism	CYP3A4 (active metabolite)	CYP2C19 (variable activation)	CYP3A4 and esterase
Half-life	7 h (parent), 8.5 h (metab)	6–8 h	7 h
Excretion	Biliary	Renal and faecal	Renal and faecal
Reversibility	Reversible	Irreversible	Irreversible

Clinical Considerations

Clopidogrel's efficacy is influenced by CYP2C19 polymorphisms, which may impair conversion to its active form and reduce platelet inhibition (Mega et al. 2009). Prasugrel provides greater potency and more consistent platelet inhibition but carries a higher bleeding risk and is contraindicated in patients with a prior history of stroke or transient ischaemic attack (Wiviott et al. 2007). Ticagrelor achieves more consistent and reversible platelet inhibition compared with clopidogrel but requires twice-daily dosing and can cause troublesome dyspnoea (Storey et al. 2010).

Doses

- **Clopidogrel:** 300 mg loading dose, followed by 75 mg once daily
- **Prasugrel:** 60 mg loading dose, then 10 mg once daily
- **Ticagrelor:** 180 mg loading dose, then 90 mg twice daily (reduced to 60 mg twice daily after one year in selected patients) (Wiviott et al. 2007; Storey et al. 2010)

9.3.3 Phosphodiesterase Inhibitors

Dipyridamole is the primary antiplatelet agent in this class. Although it has relatively weak platelet-inhibitory activity when used alone, it is often prescribed in combination with aspirin to reduce thromboembolic risk, particularly in patients with cerebrovascular disease (Diener et al. 1996).

Uses

Dipyridamole is used most commonly for secondary prevention of ischaemic stroke, usually as part of a fixed-dose combination with low-dose aspirin (Diener et al. 1996). It may also be employed in the management of peripheral arterial disease and coronary artery disease, although these are less common indications. Intravenously, dipyridamole is occasionally used as a vasodilator during pharmacologic cardiac stress testing, and it has a role in the management of pulmonary hypertension in select cases.

Mechanism of Action

Dipyridamole inhibits platelet aggregation through two primary mechanisms. First, it blocks phosphodiesterase enzymes, leading to increased intracellular cAMP levels in platelets. Elevated cAMP interferes with calcium signalling pathways essential for platelet activation. Second, it inhibits cellular reuptake of adenosine into platelets and endothelial cells. The resulting rise in extracellular adenosine stimulates adenosine receptors, promoting further cAMP accumulation and causing vasodilation. Together, these mechanisms contribute to its antiplatelet and vasodilatory effects (Rosenkranz et al. 2003).

Pharmacokinetics

Dipyridamole is available in both oral and intravenous formulations. It has moderate oral bioavailability (~50%) due to significant first-pass hepatic metabolism. The drug is highly protein bound (~99%) and is metabolised primarily in the liver via glucuronidation. Its elimination half-life is approximately 10 h, and it is excreted mainly via the biliary route with minimal renal clearance (Cocco and Chu 2021).

Side Effects

The most commonly reported adverse effects include headache, flushing, dizziness, and gastrointestinal upset such as nausea, vomiting, or diarrhoea. At higher doses or with intravenous administration, dipyridamole may provoke angina or arrhythmias, including bradycardia and ventricular tachyarrhythmias. Musculoskeletal discomfort and hepatobiliary effects, such as a potential predisposition to gallstone formation, have also been observed (Rosenkranz et al. 2003).

Other Clinical Notes

Dipyridamole is most effective when combined with aspirin in secondary stroke prevention (Diener et al. 1996). In cases of overdose or exaggerated vasodilatory response (e.g. hypotension or tachycardia), treatment with aminophylline or caffeine may be considered, as these agents antagonise adenosine receptors and reverse dipyridamole's pharmacologic effects (Cocco and Chu 2021).

9.3.4 GP IIb/IIIa Inhibitors

This drug class comprises potent intravenous antiplatelet agents that inhibit the final common pathway of platelet aggregation. Notable agents include Abciximab, Tirofiban, and Eptifibatide, with Abciximab being the most established and historically significant (Valgimigli 2009).

Uses

GP IIb/IIIa inhibitors are used primarily in high-risk patients undergoing Percutaneous Coronary Intervention (PCI) to reduce the risk of acute thrombotic complications such as stent thrombosis. They may also be employed in cases of unstable angina or Non-ST Elevation Myocardial Infarction (NSTEMI), particularly in those with large thrombus burden or ongoing ischaemia despite conventional antiplatelet therapy (Kastrati et al. 2006). Their role in STEMI is limited but may be considered in select patients undergoing primary PCI or in bail-out scenarios (e.g. no-reflow phenomenon) (De Luca et al. 2012).

Mechanism of Action

Abciximab is a monoclonal antibody fragment that binds irreversibly to the glycoprotein IIb/IIIa receptor on activated platelets. This receptor is the final site where fibrinogen and von Willebrand factor bind to crosslink platelets, enabling aggregation. By blocking this receptor, Abciximab prevents fibrinogen-mediated platelet bridging and effectively inhibits platelet aggregation, even in the presence of strong pro-thrombotic stimuli such as ADP or thromboxane A_2. The agent also exhibits partial affinity for vitronectin receptors on endothelial and smooth muscle cells, which may contribute to its pharmacodynamic profile (Valgimigli 2009).

Pharmacokinetics

Abciximab is administered intravenously and exerts an immediate onset of action. Although its plasma half-life is short (approximately 10 min), it binds tightly to platelet receptors, resulting in sustained antiplatelet activity for up to 48 h after discontinuation. Clearance occurs rapidly from plasma, but clinical effect persists due to receptor-bound drug (Valgimigli 2009).

Side Effects

The most significant adverse effect is bleeding, particularly at vascular access sites or within the gastrointestinal tract. Thrombocytopenia is another important complication and may present either acutely or in a delayed fashion. Hypersensitivity reactions, although rare, can occur due to its murine antibody component (Kastrati et al. 2006).

Other Clinical Notes

Abciximab is the Fab fragment of a chimeric human-murine monoclonal antibody, and its irreversible receptor binding differentiates it from the reversible small-molecule inhibitors like Tirofiban and Eptifibatide. Given the bleeding risk, close monitoring is essential during and after administration. Notably, oral GP IIb/IIIa inhibitors were evaluated in trials but were associated with increased mortality and have since been withdrawn from clinical use (De Luca et al. 2012) (Table 9.9).

Table 9.9 Comparison of antiplatelet agents

Drug Class	Examples	Mechanism of Action	Route	Common Side Effects	Reversal / Notes
COX Inhibitors	Aspirin	Irreversible inhibition of COX-1 → ↓ thromboxane A2 synthesis → ↓ platelet activation	Oral	Gastric irritation, GI bleeding, bronchospasm, tinnitus	No specific reversal; platelet transfusion may help
ADP Receptor (P2Y12) Inhibitors	Clopidogrel, Prasugrel, Ticagrelor	Inhibit P2Y12 ADP receptor → ↓ platelet aggregation	Oral	Bleeding (GI, dermal), dyspnoea (ticagrelor), rash	No antidote for clopidogrel/ prasugrel; Ticagrelor partially reversible with platelet transfusion
GP IIb/IIIa Inhibitors	Abciximab, Tirofiban, Eptifibatide	Inhibit GP IIb/IIIa receptor → prevent fibrinogen binding → ↓ aggregation	IV only	Bleeding (esp. GI), thrombocytopenia	Short half-life; platelet transfusion may reverse effect
Phosphodiesterase Inhibitors	Dipyridamole	Inhibits PDE → ↑ cAMP → ↓ platelet aggregation. Also blocks adenosine reuptake	Oral, IV	Headache, flushing, GI upset, hypotension	Overdose reversed with aminophylline or caffeine

Conflicts of Interest The authors have no conflicts of interest to declare that are relevant to the content of this chapter.

References

Ageno, W., Gallus, A.S., Wittkowsky, A., Crowther, M., Hylek, E.M. and Palareti, G., 2012. Oral anticoagulant therapy: Antithrombotic Therapy and Prevention of Thrombosis, 9th ed: American College of Chest Physicians Evidence-Based Clinical Practice Guidelines. *Chest*, 141(2 Suppl), pp.e44S–e88S. https://doi.org/10.1378/chest.11-2292. (PMID: 22315269)

Albaladejo, P., Samama, C.M., Sié, P., Samama, J., Marret, E., Collet, J.P., Godier, A., Rosencher, N., Steib, A., Pernod, G. and Llau, J.V., 2011. Management of antiplatelet therapy for non-elective invasive procedures or bleeding complications: proposals from the GIHP and GFHT. *Archives of Cardiovascular Diseases*, 104(12), pp.669–676. https://doi.org/10.1016/j.acvd.2011.09.001.

Antithrombotic Trialists' (ATT) Collaboration, 2002. Collaborative meta-analysis of randomised trials of antiplatelet therapy for prevention of death, myocardial infarction, and stroke in high-risk patients. *BMJ*, 324(7329), pp.71–86. https://doi.org/10.1136/bmj.324.7329.71. (PMID: 11786451)

Burger, W., Chemnitius, J.M., Kneissl, G.D. and Rücker, G., 2005. Low-dose aspirin for secondary cardiovascular prevention—risks after perioperative withdrawal vs bleeding with continuation: review and meta-analysis. *Journal of Internal Medicine*, 257(5), pp.399–414. https://doi.org/10.1111/j.1365-2796.2005.01477.x.

Chen, A., Stecker, E. and Ballew, N.G., 2020. Direct oral anticoagulant use: a practical guide to common clinical challenges. *Journal of Blood Medicine*, 11, pp.379–390. https://doi.org/10.2147/JBM.S256550. (PMID: 33177818)

Cocco, G. and Chu, D., 2021. Dipyridamole. In: *StatPearls* [Internet]. Treasure Island (FL): StatPearls Publishing. Available at: https://www.ncbi.nlm.nih.gov/books/NBK554455/ [Accessed 2 September 2025].

Connolly, S.J., Ezekowitz, M.D., Yusuf, S., Eikelboom, J., Oldgren, J., Parekh, A., Pogue, J., Reilly, P.A., Themeles, E., Varrone, J., Wang, S., Alings, M., Xavier, D., Zhu, J., Diaz, R., Lewis, B.S., Darius, H., Diener, H.C., Joyner, C.D., Wallentin, L. and RE-LY Steering Committee and Investigators, 2009. Dabigatran versus warfarin in patients with atrial fibrillation. *New England Journal of Medicine*, 361(12), pp.1139–1151. https://doi.org/10.1056/NEJMoa0905561. (PMID: 19717844)

CRASH-2 Trial Collaborators, 2010. Effects of tranexamic acid on death, vascular occlusive events, and transfusion in trauma with significant haemorrhage: randomized, placebo-controlled trial. *The Lancet*, 376(9734), pp.23–32. https://doi.org/10.1016/S0140-6736(10)60835-5. (PMID: 20554319)

De Luca, G., Verdoia, M. and Suryapranata, H., 2012. Benefits of small molecules vs abciximab in STEMI treated with primary PCI: meta-analysis of randomized trials. *Thrombosis and Haemostasis*, 107(2), pp.282–289. https://doi.org/10.1160/TH11-07-0499.

Diener, H.C., Cunha, L., Forbes, C., Sivenius, J., Smets, P. and Lowenthal, A., 1996. European Stroke Prevention Study 2: dipyridamole and acetylsalicylic acid in secondary prevention of stroke. *Journal of the Neurological Sciences*, 143(1–2), pp.1–13. https://doi.org/10.1016/S0022-510X(96)00308-5. (PMID: 8981292)

Estcourt, L.J., Birchall, J., Allard, S., Bassey, S.J., Hersey, P., Kerr, J.P., Mumford, A.D., Stanworth, S.J., Tinegate, H., Cardigan, R., Plews, D. and Llewelyn, C.A., 2017. Guidelines for the use of platelet transfusions. *British Journal of Haematology*, 176(3), pp.365–394. https://doi.org/10.1111/bjh.14423. (PMID: 27861752)

Hensley, M.K., Patel, N.J., Barrett, C.D. and Spinella, P.C., 2021. Fibrinogen concentrate for the treatment of critical bleeding. *Transfusion*, 61(Suppl 1), pp.S36–S47. https://doi.org/10.1111/trf.16561.

Hirsh, J. and Raschke, R., 2004. Heparin and low-molecular-weight heparin: Seventh ACCP Conference on Antithrombotic and Thrombolytic Therapy. *Chest*, 126(3 Suppl), pp.188S–203S. https://doi.org/10.1378/chest.126.3_suppl.188S. (PMID: 15383473)

Hofer, S., Weinzierl, M., Leichtle, A., Göbel, B., Kraschl, J., Moldovan, A. and Spreitzer, I., 2021. Management of coagulopathy in bleeding patients: FFP, cryoprecipitate and factor concentrates. *Seminars in Thrombosis and Hemostasis*, 47(6), pp.565–575. https://doi.org/10.1055/s-0041-1730810. (PMID: 34252062)

Hofer, S., Prüller, F., Jauk, V., Kleber, C., Saxer, F., Görlinger, K. and Innerhofer, P., 2022. The role of fibrinogen and fibrinogen concentrate in obstetric haemorrhage: a narrative review. *Anaesthesia Critical Care & Pain Medicine*, 41(6), p.101135. https://doi.org/10.1016/j.accpm.2022.101135. (PMID: 36542839 / PMCID: PMC9794135)

Horlocker, T.T., Vandermeulen, E., Kopp, S.L., Gogarten, W., Leffert, L.R. and Benzon, H.T., 2018. Regional anesthesia in the patient receiving antithrombotic or thrombolytic therapy: ASRA evidence-based guidelines (4th ed.). *Regional Anesthesia and Pain Medicine*, 43(3), pp.263–309. https://doi.org/10.1097/AAP.0000000000000763. (PMID: 29533317)

Hunt, B.J., Allard, S., Keeling, D., Norfolk, D., Stanworth, S.J. and Pendry, K., 2015. A practical guideline for the haematological management of major haemorrhage. *British Journal of Haematology*, 170(6), pp.788–803. https://doi.org/10.1111/bjh.13580.

Jacobs, M.R., Good, C.E., Yomtovian, R., Robitaille, R., Benjamin, R.J., Wagner, S.J., Drew, W.L., Young, C., Brecher, M.E. and Dumont, L.J., 2011. Detection of bacterial contamination in prestorage culture–negative apheresis platelets using a rapid detection system. *Transfusion*, 51(12), pp.2573–2582. https://doi.org/10.1111/j.1537-2995.2011.03184.x. (PMID: 21658033)

Johnson, J.A., Gong, L., Whirl-Carrillo, M., Gage, B.F., Scott, S.A., Stein, C.M., Anderson, J.L., Kimmel, S.E., Lee, M.T., Pirmohamed, M., Wadelius, M., Klein, T.E. and Altman, R.B., 2011. CPIC guidelines for CYP2C9 and VKORC1 genotypes and warfarin dosing. *Clinical Pharmacology & Therapeutics*, 90(4), pp.625–629. https://doi.org/10.1038/clpt.2011.185. (PMID: 21900891)

Kastrati, A., Mehilli, J., Neumann, F.J., Dotzer, F., ten Berg, J.M., Bollwein, H., Graf, I., Ibrahim, M., Pache, J., Seyfarth, M., Dirschinger, J. and Schömig, A., 2006. Abciximab in ACS patients undergoing PCI after clopidogrel pretreatment: ISAR-REACT 2 randomized trial. *JAMA*, 295(13), pp.1531–1538. https://doi.org/10.1001/jama.295.13.joc60034. (PMID: 16537725)

Keeling, D., Baglin, T., Tait, C., Watson, H., Perry, D., Baglin, C., Kitchen, S., Makris, M. and British Committee for Standards in Haematology, 2011. Guidelines on oral anticoagulation with warfarin—4th ed. *British Journal of Haematology*, 154(3), pp.311–324. https://doi.org/10.1111/j.1365-2141.2011.08753.x. (PMID: 21592016)

Kietaibl, S., Ferrandis, R., Godier, A., Llau, J.V., Samama, C.M., Van der Linden, P., Vercueil, A., Kozek-Langenecker, S., Thienpont, E., Desmet, M. and Faraoni, D., 2022. Regional anaesthesia in patients on antithrombotic drugs: Joint ESAIC/ESRA guidelines. *European Journal of Anaesthesiology*, 39(1), pp.100–132. https://doi.org/10.1097/EJA.0000000000001619. (PMID: 34817791)

Kim, K.S., 2020. Perioperative management of patients receiving non–vitamin K antagonist oral anticoagulants. *Anesthesia & Analgesia*, 130(4), pp.780–789. https://doi.org/10.1213/ANE.0000000000004562. (PMID: 32102052)

Kitchen, S., Iampietro, R., Woolley, A.M., Preston, F.E. and Jennings, I., 1999. Anti-Xa monitoring during unfractionated heparin therapy. *British Journal of Haematology*, 106(1), pp.288–289. https://doi.org/10.1046/j.1365-2141.1999.01507.x.

Kozek-Langenecker, S.A., Ahmed, A.B., Afshari, A., Albaladejo, P., Aldecoa, C., Barauskas, G., de Robertis, E., Faraoni, D., Filipescu, D.C., Fries, D., Görlinger, K., Haas, T., Ickx, B., Jacob, M., Lance, M.D., Llau, J., Mallett, S., Rahe-Meyer, N., Samama, C.M., Smith, A., Solomon, C., Van der Linden, P., Wikkelsø, A. and Wouters, P., 2017. Management of severe perioperative bleeding: guidelines from the European Society of Anaesthesiology. *European Journal of Anaesthesiology*, 34(6), pp.332–395. https://doi.org/10.1097/EJA.0000000000000630.

Leal-Noval, S.R., Muñoz, M., Asensio, Á., de la Llana, R.A., Ferrandis, R., García-Erce, J.A., Llau, J.V., Quintana-Díaz, M., Serrano-Trenas, J.A. and Trenor, A., 2025. Perioperative coagulation management and blood conservation: consensus and recommendations of the Spanish Society of Anaesthesiology and Critical Care. *Medicina Intensiva*, 49(2), pp.115–131. https://doi.org/10.1016/j.medin.2024.08.003. (PMID: 39842094 / PMCID: PMC11841953)

Levine, G.N., Bates, E.R., Bittl, J.A., Brindis, R.G., Fihn, S.D., Fleisher, L.A., Granger, C.B., Lange, R.A., Mack, M.J., Mauri, L., Mehran, R., Moussa, I.D., Mukherjee, D., Newby, L.K., O'Gara, P.T., Sabik, J.F., Smith, P.K. and Smith, S.C., 2016. 2016 ACC/AHA focused update on duration of dual antiplatelet therapy in CAD. *Journal of the American College of Cardiology*, 68(10), pp.1082–1115. https://doi.org/10.1016/j.jacc.2016.03.513. (PMID: 27036918)

Levy, J.H., Ageno, W., Chan, N.C., Crowther, M., Verhamme, P. and Weitz, J.I., 2018. When and how to use antidotes for reversal of DOACs: guidance from the SSC of the ISTH. *Journal of Thrombosis and Haemostasis*, 14(3), pp.623–627. https://doi.org/10.1111/jth.13227.

Mega, J.L., Close, S.L., Wiviott, S.D., Shen, L., Hockett, R.D., Brandt, J.T., Walker, J.R., Antman, E.M., Macias, W., Braunwald, E. and Sabatine, M.S., 2009. Cytochrome P-450 polymorphisms and response to clopidogrel. *New England Journal of Medicine*, 360(4), pp.354–362. https://doi.org/10.1056/NEJMoa0809171. (PMID: 19106084)

Mueck, W., Stampfuss, J., Kubitza, D. and Becka, M., 2014. Clinical pharmacokinetic and pharmacodynamic profile of rivaroxaban. *Clinical Pharmacokinetics*, 53(1), pp.1–16. https://doi.org/10.1007/s40262-013-0100-7. (PMID: 23999934)

Naidech, A.M., Jovanovic, B., Wartenberg, K.E., Parra, A., Ostapkovich, N., Connolly, E.S. and Mayer, S.A., 2008. Packed red blood cell transfusion causes greater haemoglobin rise at a lower starting haemoglobin in subarachnoid haemorrhage. *Neurocritical Care*, 9(2), pp.198–203. https://doi.org/10.1007/s12028-008-9062-7. (PMID: 18542851)

O'Shaughnessy, D.F., Atterbury, C., Bolton Maggs, P., Murphy, M., Thomas, D., Yates, S. and Williamson, L.M., 2004. Guidelines for the use of fresh-frozen plasma, cryoprecipitate and cryosupernatant. *British Journal of Haematology*, 126(1), pp.11–28. https://doi.org/10.1111/j.1365-2141.2004.04972.x. (PMID: 15198728)

Patel, M.R., Mahaffey, K.W., Garg, J., Pan, G., Singer, D.E., Hacke, W., Breithardt, G., Halperin, J.L., Hankey, G.J., Piccini, J.P., Becker, R.C., Nessel, C.C., Paolini, J.F., Berkowitz, S.D., Fox, K.A.A. and Califf, R.M., 2011. Rivaroxaban versus warfarin in nonvalvular atrial fibrillation. *New England Journal of Medicine*, 365(10), pp.883–891. https://doi.org/10.1056/NEJMoa1009638. (PMID: 21830957)

Patel, J.P., Roberts, L.N. and Arya, R., 2017. Anticoagulating obese patients in the modern era. *British Journal of Haematology*, 177(2), pp.191–207. https://doi.org/10.1111/bjh.14577.

Patrono, C. and Baigent, C., 2014. Aspirin, the heart, and the brain. *Circulation Research*, 114(7), pp.1058–1073. https://doi.org/10.1161/CIRCRESAHA.114.302770. (PMID: 24625788)

Patrono, C. and Baigent, C., 2019. Role of aspirin in primary prevention of cardiovascular disease. *Nature Reviews Cardiology*, 16(11), pp.675–686. https://doi.org/10.1038/s41569-019-0245-y. (PMID: 31142846)

Pollack, C.V., Reilly, P.A., Eikelboom, J., Glund, S., Verhamme, P., Bernstein, R.A., Dubiel, R., Huisman, M.V., Hylek, E.M., Kamphuisen, P.W., Kreuzer, J., Levy, J.H., Sellke, F.W., Stangier, J., Steiner, T., Wang, B., Young, L., Weitz, J.I. and RE-VERSE AD Investigators, 2015. Idarucizumab for dabigatran reversal. *New England Journal of Medicine*, 373(6), pp.511–520. https://doi.org/10.1056/NEJMoa1502000.

Roberts, I., 2015. Mechanism of action of tranexamic acid in bleeding trauma patients: exploratory analysis of CRASH-2 data. *Critical Care*, 19(1), p.87. https://doi.org/10.1186/s13054-015-0790-1.

Rosenkranz, A.C., Woods, R.L., Dusting, G.J. and Ritchie, R.H., 2003. Antihypertrophic actions of the natriuretic peptides in adult rat cardiomyocytes: importance of cyclic GMP-dependent protein kinase. *Cardiovascular Research*, 57(2), pp. 515–522.

Samama, C.M., 2008. Prothrombin complex concentrates: a brief review. *European Journal of Anaesthesiology*, 25(9), pp.784–789. https://doi.org/10.1017/S0265021508004520. (PMID: 18538049)

Sarode, R., Milling, T.J., Refaai, M.A., Mangione, A., Schneider, A., Durn, B.L., Goldstein, J.N., Huang, D.T., Pollack, C.V., Jr., and 4F-PCC Hemorrhage Study Group, 2013. Efficacy and safety of a 4-factor PCC in VKA-treated patients with major bleeding: randomized, plasma-controlled phase IIIb study. *Circulation*, 128(11), pp.1234–1243. https://doi.org/10.1161/CIRCULATIONAHA.113.002283.

Schiffer, C.A., Bohlke, K., Delaney, M., Hume, H., Magdalinski, A.J., McCullough, J.J., Omel, J.L., Rainey, J.M., Rebulla, P., Rowley, S.D., Waller, E.K. and Anderson, K.C., 2018. Platelet transfusion for patients with cancer: ASCO Clinical Practice Guideline Update. *Journal of Clinical Oncology*, 36(3), pp.283–299. https://doi.org/10.1200/JCO.2017.76.1734.

Schüpke, S., Neumann, F.J., Menichelli, M., Mayer, K., Bernlochner, I., Wöhrle, J., Richardt, G., Liebetrau, C., Witzenbichler, B., Antoniucci, D., ten Berg, J.M., Hengstenberg, C., Jacobshagen, C., Seyfarth, M., Abdel-Wahab, M., Smits, P.C., Schunkert, H. and Kastrati, A., 2019. Ticagrelor or prasugrel in patients with acute coronary syndromes. *New England Journal of Medicine*, 381(16), pp.1524–1534. https://doi.org/10.1056/NEJMoa1908973.

Stangier, J., Rathgen, K., Stähle, H. and Mazur, D., 2007. Influence of renal impairment on the PK/PD of oral dabigatran etexilate: open-label, parallel-group study. *Clinical Pharmacokinetics*, 46(9), pp.693–705. https://doi.org/10.2165/00003088-200746090-00003. (PMID: 17655343)

Storey, R.F., Becker, R.C., Harrington, R.A., Husted, S., James, S.K., Cools, F., Steg, P.G., Khurmi, N.S., Emanuelsson, H., Cooper, A., Cairns, R., Cannon, C.P. and Wallentin, L., 2010. Characterization of dyspnoea in PLATO patients treated with ticagrelor or clopidogrel. *Circulation*, 122(10), pp.1184–1192. https://doi.org/10.1161/CIRCULATIONAHA.109.927988. (PMID: 20805430)

Treleaven, J., Gennery, A., Marsh, J., Norfolk, D., Page, L., Parker, A., Saran, F. and Thurston, J., 2011. Guidelines on the use of irradiated blood components (BCSH Blood Transfusion Task Force). *British Journal of Haematology*, 152(1), pp.35–51. https://doi.org/10.1111/j.1365-2141.2010.08444.x.

Valgimigli, M., 2009. Abciximab: a reappraisal of its use in coronary care. *European Heart Journal*, 30(3), pp.256–265. https://doi.org/10.1093/eurheartj/ehn547. (PMID: 19036771)

Valgimigli, M., Bueno, H., Byrne, R.A., Collet, J.P., Costa, F., Jeppsson, A., Jüni, P., Kastrati, A., Knuuti, J., Kristensen, S.D., Moliterno, D.J., Neumann, F.J., Richter, D., Siegbahn, A., Stefanini, G.G., Storey, R.F. and Windecker, S., 2018. 2017 ESC focused update on dual antiplatelet therapy in CAD (with EACTS). *European Heart Journal*, 39(3), pp.213–260. https://doi.org/10.1093/eurheartj/ehx419. (PMID: 28886622)

van de Watering, L.M.G., 2011. Red cell storage and prognosis. *Vox Sanguinis*, 100(1), pp.36–45. https://doi.org/10.1111/j.1423-0410.2010.01441.x. (PMID: 21175653)

Wallentin, L., Becker, R.C., Budaj, A., Cannon, C.P., Emanuelsson, H., Held, C., Horrow, J., Husted, S., James, S., Katus, H., Mahaffey, K.W., Scirica, B.M., Skene, A., Steg, P.G., Storey, R.F., Harrington, R.A., Freij, A. and Thorsén, M., 2009. Ticagrelor versus clopidogrel in ACS (PLATO). *New England Journal of Medicine*, 361(11), pp.1045–1057. https://doi.org/10.1056/NEJMoa0904327. (PMID: 19717846)

Warkentin, T.E. and Greinacher, A., 2004. Heparin-induced thrombocytopenia: recognition, treatment, and prevention (Seventh ACCP). *Chest*, 126(3 Suppl), pp.311S–337S. https://doi.org/10.1378/chest.126.3_suppl.311S. (PMID: 15383477)

Weitz, J.I., 1997. Low-molecular-weight heparins. *New England Journal of Medicine*, 337(10), pp.688–698. https://doi.org/10.1056/NEJM199709043371007. (PMID: 9278469)

Wiviott, S.D., Braunwald, E., McCabe, C.H., Montalescot, G., Ruzyllo, W., Gottlieb, S., Neumann, F.J., Ardissino, D., De Servi, S., Murphy, S.A., Riesmeyer, J., Weerakkody, G., Gibson, C.M. and Antman, E.M., 2007. Prasugrel versus clopidogrel in ACS (TRITON-TIMI 38). *New England Journal of Medicine*, 357(20), pp.2001–2015. https://doi.org/10.1056/NEJMoa0706482. (PMID: 17982182)

WOMAN Trial Collaborators, 2017. Effect of early tranexamic acid on mortality, hysterectomy and morbidities in postpartum haemorrhage: international randomized double-blind trial. *The Lancet*, 389(10084), pp.2105–2116. https://doi.org/10.1016/S0140-6736(17)30638-4. (PMID: 28456509)

Anaesthesiology Drugs 10

10.1 Intravenous Anaesthetic Agents

About

Intravenous (IV) induction agents are a foundational element of modern anaesthetic practice, enabling rapid and controlled onset of unconsciousness at the commencement of general anaesthesia. The choice of induction agent is tailored to the clinical context, taking into account factors such as cardiovascular stability, comorbidities, surgical urgency, and anticipated airway difficulty. An ideal IV induction agent would produce smooth, rapid anaesthesia (within one arm–brain circulation time), exhibit haemodynamic stability, possess favourable pharmacokinetic and pharmacodynamic profiles, and minimise adverse respiratory or neurological effects. Although no agent fulfils all these criteria perfectly, an informed selection allows the anaesthetist to individualise care to optimise patient safety and procedural success (Dinis-Oliveira 2018).

Historical Context

The evolution of intravenous induction agents reflects changing priorities in anaesthetic pharmacology. Thiopentone, introduced in 1934, was the first barbiturate used for induction and dominated practice for decades due to its rapid onset and neuroprotective properties (Dundee 1984). Despite its historical importance, its use has waned due to cumulative effects, prolonged recovery, and risk of administration errors—particularly its similarity in appearance to certain antibiotics like cefazolin. Etomidate gained popularity for its cardiovascular stability but fell out of favour due to adrenal suppression via inhibition of 11β-hydroxylase, particularly in critically ill patients where it was associated with increased mortality (Valk and Struys 2021). Its use is now largely limited to select high-risk scenarios. Ketamine, first synthesised in the 1960s, is experiencing a resurgence due to its unique pharmacological profile. It provides profound analgesia, preserves airway reflexes, and maintains cardiovascular stability, making it ideal for trauma and haemodynamically unstable patients

G. Browne, *PharmacologyPro*, https://doi.org/10.1007/978-3-032-10227-0_10

(Morris et al. 2009). Beyond anaesthesia, it is increasingly used in chronic pain and psychiatric care. Propofol, introduced in the 1980s, has become the induction agent of choice in most elective anaesthetic settings. It offers rapid onset, smooth emergence, antiemetic effects, and a favourable recovery profile, though caution is warranted in haemodynamically compromised patients due to its vasodilatory effects (Dinis-Oliveira 2018).

Arm–Brain Circulation Time

The arm–brain circulation time is the interval between IV drug administration and its arrival at the cerebral cortex—typically 20–30 s in healthy adults (Dinis-Oliveira 2018). This concept underpins the pharmacodynamic suitability of induction agents, which should ideally produce anaesthesia coinciding with this timeframe to facilitate a rapid, smooth transition from Stage I (analgesia) to Stage III (surgical anaesthesia), while avoiding the undesirable features of Stage II (excitement), such as involuntary movement, breath-holding, and laryngospasm.

Summary

The landscape of IV induction agents continues to evolve, driven by improvements in safety, pharmacology, and clinical outcomes. While propofol remains the dominant agent in most high-income countries, ketamine and thiopentone retain important roles in specific clinical situations. Mastery of the pharmacological properties and appropriate application of these agents is essential for all anaesthesia practitioners (Tables 10.1 and 10.2).

Table 10.1 Clinical considerations in selection

Clinical context	Preferred Agent(s)	Rationale
Elective day-case GA	Propofol	Rapid onset, antiemetic, smooth emergence
Haemodynamically unstable (e.g. trauma)	Ketamine	Maintains BP and HR, bronchodilator
Neurosurgery / Raised ICP	Thiopentone, Propofol	Reduces cerebral metabolic demand and ICP
Cardiac surgery / ICU	Etomidate (selective use)	Haemodynamic stability (with caution re: adrenal suppression)
Obstetric anaesthesia	Propofol (modern practice)	Avoid thiopentone errors; better maternal recovery profile
Status epilepticus	Propofol, Thiopentone	Potent anticonvulsants
TIVA / Total IV Anaesthesia	Propofol (± Remifentanil)	Predictable offset, antiemetic effect

Table 10.2 Comparison of common intravenous induction agents

Drug	Mechanism of action	Haemodynamic effects	Respiratory effects	Neurological effects	Other features	Common uses
Propofol	GABA-A agonist (↑ Cl^- channel activity)	↓ SVR, ↓ BP, ↓ myocardial contractility	Dose-dependent respiratory depression; apnoea common	↓ CBF, ↓ $CMRO_2$, ↓ ICP; EEG suppression; non-epileptogenic despite myoclonic movements	Anti-emetic; pain on injection; green urine possible	Induction & maintenance of anaesthesia, sedation, refractory nausea, status epilepticus
Ketamine	NMDA antagonist; inhibits catecholamine reuptake	↑ BP, ↑ HR, ↑ CO (sympathomimetic); caution in IHD	Preserved RR and airway reflexes; bronchodilation	↑ CBF, ↑ $CMRO_2$, ↑ ICP; dissociative anaesthesia; emergence delirium possible	Analgesic; multiple routes (IV, IM, oral, nasal, rectal); contraindicated in eye trauma, porphyria	Haemodynamic instability, trauma, asthma, sedation, analgesia
Thiopentone	GABA-A agonist (↑ Cl^- conductance)	↓ SVR, ↓ BP; may cause myocardial depression	Dose-dependent depression; apnoea	↓ CBF, ↓ $CMRO_2$, ↓ ICP; burst suppression on EEG; porphyrogenic	Used in neuroanaesthesia; may precipitate bronchospasm; long context-sensitive half-life with infusions	Induction, neuroprotection, status epilepticus, previously used in obstetrics
Etomidate	GABA-A agonist	Minimal effect on BP & HR; haemodynamically stable	Minimal respiratory depression	↓ CBF, ↓ $CMRO_2$, ↓ ICP	Inhibits 11β-hydroxylase → adrenal suppression; myoclonus; pain on injection	Induction in haemodynamically unstable patients (limited by adrenal suppression in ICU use)

10.1.1 Propofol

Class: Intravenous general anaesthetic agent; alkylphenol derivative.

Uses

Propofol is widely used for the induction and maintenance of general anaesthesia due to its rapid onset and short duration of action. It is also employed for procedural sedation in settings such as endoscopy and bronchoscopy, short-term sedation in the intensive care unit (ICU), and for the treatment of refractory status epilepticus (Parviainen et al. 2007). At low doses, it has antiemetic properties and can be used to manage refractory postoperative nausea and vomiting (Borgeat and Stirnemann 1998). Its neuroprotective and anticonvulsant properties make it suitable in specific neurosurgical and seizure-related contexts (Parviainen et al. 2007).

Mechanism of Action

Propofol acts primarily by potentiating the inhibitory neurotransmitter γ-aminobutyric acid (GABA) at the GABA-A receptor. By binding to an allosteric site on the receptor, it increases the duration of chloride channel opening, resulting in hyperpolarisation of the post-synaptic membrane and CNS depression. The clinical effects include hypnosis, amnesia, sedation, and loss of consciousness (Garcia et al. 2010) (Table 10.3).

Pharmacodynamics / Effects

Propofol produces significant cardiovascular depression through dose-dependent vasodilation, resulting in reduced systemic vascular resistance, preload, and afterload. It also exhibits mild negative inotropy, and bradycardia or even asystole may occur via vagal stimulation. Respiratory depression is common, particularly after a bolus dose, often leading to apnoea (Sahinovic et al. 2018). Despite this, it also has bronchodilatory effects and is well tolerated in asthmatic patients. Within the CNS,

Table 10.3 Pharmacokinetics

Property	Details
Administration	IV only; available in 1% (10 mg/mL) and 2% (20 mg/mL) lipid emulsion
Onset	30–60 s
Duration	4–8 min (after single bolus)
Volume of distribution	~2–10 L/kg (large due to lipophilicity)
Protein Binding	~99%
Metabolism	Hepatic (glucuronidation and hydroxylation); extrahepatic metabolism (lung)
Elimination half-life	Terminal half-life 1–2 h (bolus); 4–30 h (context-dependent infusion)
Excretion	Renally as inactive metabolites

Table 10.4 Doses of propofol

Indication	Dose
Induction (adults)	1.5–2.5 mg/kg IV bolus
Induction (children)	2–3 mg/kg IV bolus
Sedation (procedural)	0.5–1 mg/kg bolus, then 25–75 μg/kg/min infusion
Maintenance (TIVA)	100–150 μg/kg/min (adult); 200–300 μg/kg/min (paediatric)
Status epilepticus	1–2 mg/kg bolus, then 30–100 μg/kg/min infusion
Antiemetic	10–20 mg bolus or 10 μg/kg/min infusion

propofol reduces intracranial pressure, cerebral metabolic rate ($CMRO_2$), and cerebral blood flow, and it has anticonvulsant activity making it useful in refractory seizures, although it may cause transient myoclonic or dystonic movements that are not epileptiform (Sahinovic et al. 2018). Its antiemetic effects are thought to be mediated through receptor activity in the chemoreceptor trigger zone (Borgeat and Stirnemann 1998). Propofol may also cause green or pink discolouration of urine due to phenol metabolites, which is benign. A rare but serious complication is propofol infusion syndrome (PRIS), particularly during prolonged high-dose infusions in ICU, characterised by metabolic acidosis, rhabdomyolysis, renal failure, and cardiovascular collapse (Vasile et al. 2003).

Side Effects

The most frequent adverse effects include hypotension, bradycardia, apnoea, and injection site pain (up to 70% incidence), which may be mitigated by prior administration of lidocaine or using a larger vein (Sahinovic et al. 2018). Myoclonic or dystonic movements, though transient, can be concerning. Hypertriglyceridaemia may occur with prolonged infusion. PRIS is a rare but potentially fatal complication seen with prolonged, high-dose administration, especially in children or critically ill patients (Vasile et al. 2003).

Other Considerations

Propofol is formulated in a lipid emulsion containing egg phosphatide, soybean oil, and glycerol. While caution is often advised in patients with egg or soy allergy, true anaphylaxis is rare. As the emulsion supports bacterial growth, vials must be used within 6 h of opening. Due to PRIS risk, long-term sedation with propofol is not recommended in paediatrics (Vasile et al. 2003). Its characteristic white, milky appearance has led to its colloquial nickname, the "Milk of Amnesia." (Table 10.4).

10.1.2 Ketamine

Class

Phencyclidine derivative; dissociative anaesthetic agent (Mion 2017).

Uses

Ketamine is a versatile agent used for the induction of anaesthesia, particularly in haemodynamically unstable patients due to its cardiovascular stimulating properties. It is widely used for procedural sedation in emergency and trauma settings (e.g., burns dressings, emergency airway management), and increasingly as an adjunct or primary agent for analgesia in both acute and chronic pain, including trauma and sickle cell crises. Ketamine is valuable in rapid sequence induction (RSI), particularly in prehospital or military environments. It also plays a role in ICU and palliative care sedation, and can be used in low doses as an adjunct to spinal or epidural anaesthesia. Its potent bronchodilatory effect makes it suitable for severe asthma unresponsive to conventional therapy (Kurdi et al. 2014).

Mechanism of Action

Ketamine exerts its effects primarily through non-competitive antagonism of the N-methyl-D-aspartate (NMDA) receptor, blocking excitatory glutamate transmission and producing analgesia, amnesia, anaesthesia, and neuroplastic modulation. It also weakly stimulates μ, κ, and δ opioid receptors, contributing to analgesia. Inhibition of monoamine reuptake (dopamine, noradrenaline, serotonin) results in central sympathomimetic effects such as increased heart rate and blood pressure. Additionally, ketamine inhibits muscarinic receptors and voltage-gated calcium channels, which further contribute to its anticholinergic and analgesic profile (Mion 2017; Peltoniemi et al. 2016).

Pharmacodynamics/Effects

Ketamine typically causes an increase in heart rate, blood pressure, and cardiac output due to central sympathetic stimulation. However, in catecholamine-depleted states such as septic shock or in the elderly, myocardial depression may predominate. It has minimal respiratory depression and uniquely preserves airway reflexes and spontaneous ventilation, making it advantageous in emergency settings. As a potent bronchodilator, it is particularly useful in patients with reactive airway disease. In the CNS, ketamine raises intracranial pressure, cerebral blood flow, and $CMRO_2$, and may worsen pre-existing raised ICP. It induces a dissociative state characterised by catalepsy, analgesia, and amnesia, with the eyes open and nystagmus present. EEG patterns may mimic seizure activity despite the absence of cortical involvement. Other systemic effects include increased salivation, nausea, vomiting, raised intraocular pressure, and occasional transient elevation of liver enzymes (Peltoniemi et al. 2016; Kurdi et al. 2014) (Table 10.5).

Side Effects

Common adverse effects include emergence phenomena such as vivid hallucinations, nightmares, and confusion—typically mitigated by co-administration of

Table 10.5 Pharmacokinetics of Ketamine

Property	Details
Administration	IV, IM, oral, nasal, subcutaneous, rectal, epidural, sublingual
Bioavailability	Oral: 15–30%, Intranasal: ~45%, IM: ~90%, Epidural: ~75%
Onset	IV: 30–60 s, IM: 3–5 min, Oral: 10–30 min
Duration (IV)	5–10 min for anaesthesia, longer for analgesia
Protein binding	Low (~30%)
Metabolism	Hepatic via CYP3A4, CYP2C9, CYP2B6 to active norketamine
Excretion	Renal (mostly as conjugated inactive metabolites)
Elimination half-life	Ketamine: 2.5–3 h; Norketamine: ~12 h (longer-lasting analgesia)

Table 10.6 Ketamine Doses

Indication	Dose
Anaesthesia (IV)	1–2 mg/kg IV bolus (induction)
Anaesthesia (IM)	4–10 mg/kg IM (useful in children, uncooperative)
Analgesia	0.2–0.5 mg/kg IV bolus or infusion (5–10 μg/kg/min)
Status Asthmaticus	1–2 mg/kg IV bolus, then infusion (0.5–1 mg/kg/hr)
Sedation	0.25–0.5 mg/kg IV or 2–4 mg/kg IM

benzodiazepines (Sener et al. 2011). Excessive salivation may necessitate the use of anticholinergic agents like glycopyrrolate. Other effects include postoperative nausea and vomiting, cardiac arrhythmias in susceptible individuals, and urinary tract symptoms such as ketamine-induced cystitis with chronic misuse (Shahani et al. 2007). Its propensity to increase ICP and IOP necessitates careful patient selection (Kurdi et al. 2014).

Contraindications

Ketamine is contraindicated in patients with penetrating ocular trauma, raised intracranial pressure, or known intracranial mass lesions. It should be avoided in individuals with a history of psychosis or schizophrenia due to the risk of exacerbation (Kurdi et al. 2014). Uncontrolled hypertension, ischaemic heart disease, and porphyria are also relative contraindications.

Other Points

Ketamine is known as a drug of abuse due to its dissociative and hallucinogenic effects, although at subanaesthetic doses, it is increasingly recognised for its analgesic and opioid-sparing properties. It is unique among induction agents in that it maintains airway reflexes and haemodynamic stability (Kurdi et al. 2014). Co-administration with benzodiazepines reduces the risk of emergence delirium (Sener et al. 2011). Clinically available ketamine is a racemic mixture, while S(+)-ketamine (esketamine) offers higher potency and fewer psychotropic effects (Kurdi et al. 2014) (Table 10.6).

10.1.3 Thiopentone

Class
Barbiturate; ultra–short-acting intravenous anaesthetic agent.

Uses
Thiopentone remains a valuable agent in specific clinical settings despite its widespread replacement by newer agents like propofol. It is primarily used for the induction of general anaesthesia when rapid onset is required, particularly in neuroanaesthesia where cerebral protection is critical (Matta et al. 1995). It also serves as an effective anticonvulsant in the management of refractory status epilepticus (Govindarajan et al. 2004) and is occasionally employed in electroconvulsive therapy (ECT). Outside of medical practice, it has been controversially used in lethal injection protocols.

Mechanism of Action
Thiopentone enhances inhibitory neurotransmission through GABA-A receptor potentiation, increasing the duration of chloride channel opening, which hyperpolarises neuronal membranes and suppresses action potential generation. This results in rapid onset of unconsciousness, sedation, and anticonvulsant activity. It also inhibits excitatory neurotransmission by antagonising AMPA receptors and markedly reduces the cerebral metabolic rate ($CMRO_2$) (Matta et al. 1995).

Pharmacodynamics / Effects
Centrally, thiopentone causes a profound decrease in $CMRO_2$, cerebral blood flow, and intracranial pressure, making it ideal for neuroprotection during neurosurgical procedures (Matta et al. 1995). It produces EEG burst suppression at high doses and is effective in seizure control (Govindarajan et al. 2004), though it lacks intrinsic analgesic properties. Cardiovascular effects include dose-dependent hypotension due to decreased systemic vascular resistance, though myocardial depression is less pronounced than with propofol. Respiratory depression is common, often leading to reduced tidal volume and respiratory rate or apnoea. It does not possess bronchodilatory properties and may provoke bronchospasm or laryngospasm on emergence, particularly in patients with reactive airway disease. Thiopentone is contraindicated in porphyria, as it can precipitate acute attacks. It also induces hepatic microsomal enzymes, potentially altering the metabolism of other drugs (Butterworth and Mackey 2022) (Table 10.7).

Side Effects
Adverse effects include hypotension, apnoea, bronchospasm, and laryngospasm (Shukla et al. 2010). Paradoxical excitation or myoclonus may occur during induction. It can cause severe venous irritation, and extravasation must be avoided due to the risk of tissue necrosis. Intra-arterial injection is particularly dangerous and must be avoided (Shibata et al. 2016). In susceptible individuals, particularly the elderly or after repeated high doses, prolonged somnolence may occur. Thiopentone is an absolute contraindication in patients with acute intermittent porphyria.

Table 10.7 Pharmacokinetics of Thiopentone

Property	Details
Administration	IV (common), rectal/oral (rare in clinical use today)
Onset	<30 s (very rapid)
Duration	5–10 min after single IV dose
Protein binding	~80%
Metabolism	Hepatic (oxidation) to inactive metabolites (some converted to pentobarbitone)
Elimination	Renal
Half-life	~5–10 h (single bolus); up to 26 h post-infusion (context-sensitive)
Special features	Zero-order kinetics with prolonged infusion (saturation kinetics)
Enzyme effects	Induces CYP450 enzymes → increases metabolism of other drugs

Table 10.8 Thiopentone doses

Indication	Dose
IV Induction (adults)	3–7 mg/kg
Paediatric rectal administration	20–30 mg/kg PR (max 1 g)
Status epilepticus	100–250 mg IV boluses titrated
Neuroprotection/burst suppression	Infusion titrated to EEG target

Other Notes

First introduced in 1934, thiopentone revolutionised anaesthetic practice and became the standard IV induction agent for decades (Dundee 1984). Although largely replaced by propofol for routine induction due to its more favourable recovery profile, thiopentone remains in use in select neuroanaesthesia cases and for its anticonvulsant properties. It was historically used in obstetric anaesthesia but is now less favoured due to neonatal respiratory depression. The drug is supplied as a powder and requires reconstitution with sterile water before use. Due to its high alkalinity, thiopentone precipitates in acidic solutions and is incompatible with many other IV medications (Table 10.8).

10.1.4 Etomidate

Class

Imidazole-derived intravenous anaesthetic agent.

Uses

Etomidate is primarily used for the induction of anaesthesia, particularly in patients who are haemodynamically unstable, such as those with hypovolaemia, trauma, or poor cardiac function. Its minimal cardiovascular effects also make it suitable for critical care procedural sedation. Although it has favourable cerebral effects and was historically used in neuroanaesthesia and rapid sequence induction (RSI), its routine use has declined due to concerns about adrenal suppression and increased mortality in critically ill patients, especially those with sepsis (Hildreth et al. 2008; Vinclair et al. 2008).

Mechanism of Action

Etomidate enhances GABAergic inhibition by binding to the GABA-A receptor and increasing the frequency of chloride channel opening. This results in hyperpolarisation of neuronal membranes and suppression of neuronal activity, producing sedation and hypnosis (Renou et al. 1978).

Pharmacodynamics/Effects

Etomidate reduces cerebral blood flow, intracranial pressure, and cerebral metabolic oxygen consumption ($CMRO_2$), while preserving autoregulation—features that were once highly valued in neuroanaesthesia (Renou et al. 1978). Cardiovascular stability is its hallmark; etomidate causes minimal changes in heart rate, systemic vascular resistance, or myocardial contractility, making it especially useful in patients with cardiac compromise or haemodynamic instability. Respiratory depression is generally mild and less likely to cause apnoea compared to agents like propofol or thiopentone. However, it lacks bronchodilatory effects. Endocrinologically, etomidate inhibits the enzyme 11β-hydroxylase in the adrenal cortex, leading to decreased cortisol and aldosterone synthesis. This adrenal suppression may persist for over 24 h after a single dose and has been linked to increased mortality in septic ICU patients (Hildreth et al. 2008; Vinclair et al. 2008) (Table 10.9).

Side Effects

The most notable adverse effect of etomidate is adrenal suppression, which limits its use in critically ill patients and contraindicates its use in adrenal insufficiency or septic shock (Vinclair et al. 2008; Hildreth et al. 2008). Myoclonus is common, occurring in up to 80% of patients, and while not harmful, it may be misinterpreted as seizure activity. Pain on injection is frequently reported, along with nausea, vomiting, hiccups, and involuntary movements (Forman 2011). EEG may show seizure-like activity, although this is not typically associated with true convulsive behaviour (Forman 2011).

Other Notes

Etomidate is supplied either in a lipid emulsion or propylene glycol solution. Its haemodynamic neutrality makes it useful in trauma, cardiac tamponade, pericarditis, and severe hypovolaemia. However, it has no analgesic properties and should

Table 10.9 Etomidate pharmacokinetics

Property	Description
Route	Intravenous only
Onset	Rapid (<30 s)
Duration	3–10 min (due to redistribution)
Protein binding	~75%
Metabolism	Hepatic and plasma esterases via hydrolysis
Elimination half-life	2–5 h
Excretion	Renal and biliary

Table 10.10 Etomidate doses

Indication	Dose
Induction (adult)	0.2–0.3 mg/kg IV
Sedation	0.1 mg/kg IV (titrated)

be combined with opioids when pain relief is required. It is not recommended for continuous infusion due to prolonged adrenal suppression (Forman 2011; Vinclair et al. 2008). Caution is advised in patients with sepsis, those on long-term corticosteroids, or those with known adrenal dysfunction (Hildreth et al. 2008) (Table 10.10).

10.2 Inhalational Anaesthetic Agents

10.2.1 Volatile Agents

About

Inhalational anaesthetic agents are volatile liquids or gases delivered via vapour through a face mask, laryngeal mask airway (LMA), endotracheal tube (ETT), or tracheostomy. They are used extensively for the induction and maintenance of general anaesthesia, particularly in paediatric and ambulatory surgery. These agents are classified into two main groups: volatile agents (e.g. sevoflurane, isoflurane, desflurane, halothane), which require dedicated vaporizers, and the non-volatile gas nitrous oxide. Vaporizers enable the controlled conversion of volatile liquids into vapour for precise administration in the inspiratory gas mix.

Theories of Action

The mechanism by which inhalational agents produce anaesthesia is not fully elucidated. The Meyer–Overton hypothesis proposes that anaesthetic potency is directly proportional to lipid solubility, implying that agents dissolve into lipid membranes and perturb ion channel activity (Alkire et al. 2004). Another leading theory involves neurotransmitter modulation, whereby inhaled agents enhance inhibitory synaptic activity (e.g. through GABA-A receptor potentiation) and suppress excitatory transmission (e.g. via NMDA receptor antagonism) (Franks 2006).

Minimum Alveolar Concentration (MAC)

MAC is the alveolar concentration of a volatile anaesthetic required to prevent movement in response to a standard surgical stimulus (typically a skin incision) in 50% of patients. MAC values are age-dependent, additive across agents, and used as a clinical guide to anaesthetic depth. For example, administering 0.3 MAC nitrous oxide alongside 0.8 MAC sevoflurane yields a total of 1.1 MAC. MAC90 reflects the concentration needed to prevent movement in 90% of individuals. Studies demonstrate that MAC is determined primarily at the spinal cord level rather than the brain (Rampil 1994) (Table 10.11).

Table 10.11 Factors which affect MAC

Increased MAC	Decreased MAC
Young age	Elderly
Chronic alcohol use	Pregnancy
Hyperthermia	Acute alcohol intoxication
CNS stimulants (e.g. amphetamines)	Hypothermia
Hypernatremia	CNS depressants (e.g. opioids, benzodiazepines)
Hyperthyroidism	Hypotension
	Hyponatremia
	Hypothyroidism
	Ketamine
	Hypoxia

Partition Coefficients

Two key partition coefficients define inhalational agent behaviour:

- **Blood:Gas Partition Coefficient (BGPC)** reflects blood solubility. Agents with a low BGPC (e.g. desflurane) have rapid onset and recovery, while agents with a high BGPC (e.g. halothane) have slower kinetics due to greater blood solubility and reservoir effect (Esper et al. 2015).
- **Oil:Gas Partition Coefficient (OGPC)** reflects lipid solubility and correlates with anaesthetic potency. Higher OGPC values indicate greater lipid solubility, lower MAC, and increased potency.

Side Effects of Inhalational Agents

Inhaled agents can cause systemic toxicity. Hepatotoxicity, particularly with halothane, is well recognised: Type 1 is a mild, self-limiting elevation in liver enzymes, while Type 2 is an immune-mediated fulminant hepatitis with a mortality rate approaching 70% (Dhanasekaran et al. 2011). Nephrotoxicity has been associated with methoxyflurane (via inorganic fluoride ions) and sevoflurane (via Compound A, see below). Nitrous oxide inhibits methionine synthase by oxidising vitamin B12, which may result in bone marrow suppression, subacute combined degeneration of the spinal cord, or megaloblastic anaemia. Other adverse effects include myocardial depression, respiratory depression, and malignant hyperthermia in genetically susceptible individuals.

Compound A and Sevoflurane

Sevoflurane may degrade to Compound A when exposed to strong alkali in CO_2 absorbents like soda lime. Although nephrotoxicity has been observed in rats at concentrations >200 ppm, the highest levels reported in humans have been approximately 20 ppm, with no clinical toxicity demonstrated (Frink et al. 1992). Nonetheless, prolonged low-flow sevoflurane anaesthesia should be avoided in closed-circuit systems to reduce theoretical risk.

Summary
Volatile inhalational agents remain a fundamental component of general anaesthesia. Understanding their physicochemical properties—particularly MAC values and partition coefficients—is essential to ensure safe and effective use. Clinicians must also be familiar with specific adverse effects, contraindications, and patient-tailored considerations, particularly when combining multiple agents or managing high-risk surgical patients.

10.2.2 Nitrous Oxide

Nitrous oxide (N_2O) is a colourless, odourless gas with both anaesthetic and analgesic properties. Although a weak anaesthetic agent when used alone, it provides potent analgesia and remains widely used in obstetric, dental, and procedural contexts. Its rapid onset, ease of administration, and minimal metabolism make it valuable both as a standalone agent for short procedures and as an adjunct to volatile and intravenous anaesthetics (Knuf and Maani 2025). It is particularly useful in paediatric anaesthesia and emergency settings.

Clinical Uses
Nitrous oxide is commonly used for labour analgesia (administered as Entonox—a 50:50 pre-mixed combination of N_2O and O_2), procedural sedation (e.g. during wound closure or fracture reduction), and as an adjunct in general anaesthesia, where it enhances the speed of induction via the second gas effect and reduces the MAC of co-administered volatile agents. In paediatrics and dental anaesthesia, nitrous oxide is favoured for its rapid onset and minimal haemodynamic disturbance (Knuf and Maani 2025).

Entonox (50:50 N_2O/O_2 Mixture)
Entonox is delivered via a demand-valve system and provides rapid-onset, short-duration analgesia without requiring IV access. However, special care must be taken in its storage. At low temperatures, gas lamination can occur, with nitrous oxide potentially separating and liquefying. This stratification may cause the initial gas delivered to be nearly pure oxygen, followed by a dangerously hypoxic mixture. Cylinders should be stored horizontally at temperatures above 10 °C and inverted before use if lamination is suspected (Flook 1972).

Pharmacodynamics
Nitrous oxide has minimal cardiovascular effects, with slight myocardial depression typically offset by increased sympathetic tone. However, it does increase pulmonary vascular resistance and should be avoided in patients with pulmonary hypertension. Cerebrally, it increases cerebral blood flow, intracranial pressure, and cerebral oxygen consumption—making it unsuitable for patients with raised ICP. Respiratory effects include a mild central depressant action, with increased respiratory rate and decreased tidal volume, though minute ventilation is generally maintained.

Importantly, N_2O does not blunt the hypoxic ventilatory drive significantly. Its analgesic properties are attributed to NMDA receptor antagonism and endogenous opioid release (Knuf and Maani 2025).

Side Effects & Risks

Postoperative nausea and vomiting (PONV) is common, occurring in up to 30–50% of patients, and its use should be avoided in high-risk individuals. Bone marrow suppression may occur with chronic exposure due to inhibition of methionine synthase via vitamin B12 oxidation, leading to megaloblastic anaemia, peripheral neuropathy, and—in severe cases—subacute combined degeneration of the spinal cord (Frasca et al. 1986). Expansion of closed gas spaces is a major concern due to the high solubility of nitrous oxide in blood (34 times greater than nitrogen). N_2O rapidly diffuses into air-filled cavities, increasing volume and pressure. It is therefore contraindicated in pneumothorax, bowel obstruction, pneumocephalus, middle ear procedures, air embolism, and following intraocular gas injection (e.g. sulphur hexafluoride or perfluoropropane) (Knuf and Maani 2025). Environmental concerns are also significant. Nitrous oxide is a potent greenhouse gas with a long atmospheric lifetime, contributing to climate change. Many institutions are actively reducing its use or removing piped nitrous oxide systems in line with sustainability initiatives.

Pharmacokinetics

Nitrous oxide has a MAC of approximately 105%, making it insufficiently potent for surgical anaesthesia in isolation. Its low blood:gas partition coefficient (~0.47) confers rapid onset and offset, and it is eliminated unchanged via the lungs (Knuf and Maani 2025). It enhances the uptake of more soluble volatile agents through the second gas effect.

Summary

Nitrous oxide continues to play a role in selected anaesthetic and analgesic contexts due to its rapid onset, analgesic properties, and ease of administration. However, its limitations—including poor anaesthetic potency, risk of gas expansion in closed spaces, potential for neurotoxicity in B12-deficient patients, and its environmental impact—necessitate careful patient selection and institutional stewardship. Its future use may become increasingly restricted as sustainability efforts intensify (Table 10.12).

Table 10.12 Comparison of inhalational agents

Feature	Sevoflurane	Desflurane	Isoflurane	Halothane	Nitrous Oxide
MAC (%)	2.0	6.0	1.2	0.75	104
Blood:Gas Coefficient	0.65	0.42	1.4	2.3	0.47
Oil:Gas Coefficient	47	18.7	91	224	1.4
Onset/Offset	Moderate	Very rapid	Slow	Slow	Very rapid
Metabolism (%)	2–5%	<0.1%	0.2%	20%	0.004%
Organ Toxicity	Compound A (nephrotoxicity in animals)	Airway irritant	Airway irritant	Halothane hepatitis	Bone marrow suppression (B12 inhibition)
Effect on ICP	↓ or stable	↑	↑	↑	↑
Effect on BP	↓	↓	↓	↓	Minimal
Airway Irritation	None	Yes (pungent)	Yes (pungent)	None	None
Environmental Impact	High (Greenhouse gas)	Very high (Significant GHG)	High	High	Very high (Potent greenhouse gas)
Special Notes	Preferred agent for inhalational induction	Not used for induction due to pungency	Rarely used today	Now obsolete due to hepatitis risk	Used in Entonox; avoid in closed gas spaces

10.3 Neuromuscular Blocking Drugs

About

Neuromuscular blocking drugs (NMBs) are an essential component of modern anaesthetic and critical care practice. They are used to facilitate tracheal intubation, ensure immobility and optimal surgical exposure, and enable controlled mechanical ventilation—particularly in critical care settings such as acute respiratory distress syndrome (ARDS). These agents act at the neuromuscular junction, inhibiting signal transmission between motor nerves and skeletal muscles, leading to flaccid paralysis (Adeyinka and Senba 2024). It is crucial to recognise that neuromuscular blockers do not possess any sedative, anxiolytic, or analgesic properties. As such, they must never be administered to a conscious or inadequately anaesthetised patient. Awareness under paralysis is a rare but devastating complication, and appropriate hypnotic and analgesic cover must be ensured throughout their use (Driver et al. 2022).

Types of Neuromuscular Blockers

Neuromuscular blockers are categorised into depolarising and non-depolarising agents based on their mechanism of action. Depolarising agents mimic acetylcholine (ACh) by binding to nicotinic receptors at the neuromuscular junction, causing continuous depolarisation of the motor endplate. This persistent stimulation leads initially to muscle fasciculations, followed by desensitisation and flaccid paralysis. The sole clinically used depolarising agent is suxamethonium (succinylcholine), prized for its rapid onset and ultra-short duration, making it ideal for rapid sequence induction (Adeyinka and Senba 2024). Non-depolarising agents, by contrast, competitively inhibit the binding of ACh to nicotinic receptors without depolarising the muscle membrane. This results in dose-dependent skeletal muscle paralysis that can be reversed pharmacologically. Examples include rocuronium, vecuronium, cisatracurium, atracurium, pancuronium, and mivacurium. These agents vary in onset time, duration of action, metabolism, and organ dependency, allowing tailoring to specific patient needs and procedural durations (Adeyinka and Senba 2024).

Reversal of Blockade

Reversal of neuromuscular blockade is a key consideration at the end of surgery to ensure the return of spontaneous respiration, airway protective reflexes, and patient safety. Traditional reversal involves the use of acetylcholinesterase inhibitors, most commonly neostigmine (typically 2.5 mg IV). This agent increases acetylcholine concentration at the neuromuscular junction, overcoming receptor blockade. Because neostigmine also stimulates muscarinic receptors, it is co-administered with glycopyrronium (0.5 mg IV) to counteract bradycardia and secretions. These drugs are commonly supplied as a pre-mixed 1 mL solution. Sugammadex represents a modern, highly selective reversal agent for aminosteroidal neuromuscular blockers such as rocuronium and vecuronium. It acts via encapsulation, leading to rapid and complete reversal even after profound or deep blockade. Sugammadex has a more predictable profile than neostigmine and avoids the cholinergic side effects associated with acetylcholinesterase inhibitors, making it particularly valuable in high-risk or urgent extubation scenarios (Moss et al. 2022).

10.3.1 Non-Depolarising NMBs

Non-depolarising neuromuscular blockers (NDNMBs) are a cornerstone of anaesthetic and critical care practice. They are commonly administered to facilitate tracheal intubation, achieve skeletal muscle relaxation during surgery, and enhance synchrony with mechanical ventilation—particularly in intensive care or when neuromuscular junction transmission needs to be temporarily interrupted (Adeyinka and Senba 2024).

Mechanism of Action

NDNMBs act as competitive antagonists at the post-synaptic nicotinic acetylcholine receptors (nAChRs) located at the neuromuscular junction. By binding to the receptor without activating it, they prevent acetylcholine (ACh) from triggering depolarisation of the muscle membrane, resulting in flaccid paralysis. Clinically significant neuromuscular blockade typically requires occupancy of approximately 80–90% of these receptors (Adeyinka and Senba 2024).

Notable Agents

- **Atracurium** is a benzylisoquinolinium compound that undergoes Hofmann elimination and ester hydrolysis, allowing metabolism independent of hepatic or renal function. However, it can cause histamine release. The usual intubating dose is 0.5 mg/kg IV (Ritz 2023).
- **Cisatracurium** is a stereoisomer of atracurium with similar metabolism but without significant histamine release, making it more haemodynamically stable and preferable in high-risk patients (Doenicke et al. 1997).
- **Rocuronium** is a steroidal NMB used for both routine and rapid sequence intubation (RSI). A dose of 0.6 mg/kg is used for elective intubation, whereas 1.2 mg/kg provides onset comparable to suxamethonium. Duration of action is typically 30–60 min (Adeyinka and Senba 2024).
- **Pancuronium** is a long-acting steroidal NMB known for its vagolytic properties, which can lead to tachycardia. The standard dose is 0.1 mg/kg. Its prolonged duration makes it suitable for prolonged surgical procedures but less favourable for short cases or fast recovery (Adeyinka and Senba 2024).
- **Mivacurium** is a very short-acting benzylisoquinolinium NMB that is rapidly hydrolysed by plasma cholinesterase. While useful in brief procedures, its metabolism can be unpredictable in patients with pseudocholinesterase deficiency. Histamine release may occur at higher doses (Adeyinka and Senba 2024).

Reversal of NDNMB

Neostigmine, an acetylcholinesterase inhibitor, is the traditional reversal agent. It increases acetylcholine concentration at the neuromuscular junction, allowing it to outcompete the NDNMB. Because acetylcholine also stimulates muscarinic receptors, glycopyrronium is co-administered to mitigate side effects such as bradycardia, salivation, and bronchospasm. The two are commonly supplied in a fixed 2.5 mg:0.5 mg combination. Sugammadex is a selective reversal agent for aminosteroidal NMBs such as rocuronium and vecuronium. It acts by encapsulating the drug molecule, rendering it inactive. Sugammadex provides rapid, complete reversal even after profound blockade and does not have the cholinergic side effects associated with neostigmine. However, it is not effective against benzylisoquinolinium agents like atracurium or cisatracurium (Adeyinka and Senba 2024) (Table 10.13).

Table 10.13 Common non-depolarising neuromuscular blockers

Drug	Duration	Metabolism	Histamine release	Sugammadex reversible	Key features
Rocuronium	Intermediate	Hepatic	No	Yes	Rapid onset, RSI alternative
Vecuronium	Intermediate	Hepatic	No	Yes	Slower onset than roc
Atracurium	Intermediate	Hofmann + esterases	Yes	No	Avoid in asthma
Cisatracurium	Intermediate	Hofmann	No	No	Ideal in organ dysfunction
Pancuronium	Long	Hepatic + renal	No	No	Long cardiac procedures
Mivacurium	Short	Plasma cholinesterase	Yes	No	Rarely used

10.3.2 Depolarising NMBs

Depolarising neuromuscular blockers function by mimicking acetylcholine (ACh) at the neuromuscular junction. Unlike non-depolarising agents, these drugs initially stimulate the nicotinic ACh receptor, resulting in transient depolarisation and visible muscle fasciculations. This is followed by sustained depolarisation and receptor desensitisation, ultimately leading to flaccid paralysis. The only depolarising agent in routine clinical use is suxamethonium (also known as succinylcholine), which remains a key drug for rapid neuromuscular blockade due to its unique pharmacokinetic profile (Hager et al. 2025).

10.3.2.1 Suxamethonium

Clinical Uses

Suxamethonium is the agent of choice for rapid sequence induction (RSI) of anaesthesia, particularly in emergency settings where securing the airway quickly is critical. Its rapid onset and short duration also make it useful for short procedures requiring transient paralysis, such as electroconvulsive therapy (ECT). It is highly effective for facilitating tracheal intubation when rapid neuromuscular relaxation is required (Cook 2023).

Mechanism of Action

Suxamethonium causes a Phase I depolarising block by binding to nicotinic ACh receptors at the motor endplate, opening ion channels and causing continuous depolarisation of the muscle membrane. This results in an initial phase of fasciculations, followed by flaccid paralysis. Unlike acetylcholine, suxamethonium is not broken down by synaptic acetylcholinesterase. Instead, it remains bound to the receptor until it passively diffuses away and is metabolised by plasma cholinesterase (also known as pseudocholinesterase), allowing neuromuscular transmission to resume (Hager et al. 2025).

Table 10.14 Suxamethonium side effects

Side effect	Mechanism/Clinical relevance
Malignant Hyperthermia	Potent trigger in susceptible patients
Hyperkalaemia	Can cause life-threatening arrhythmias in at-risk patients
Increased Intraocular Pressure	Avoid in open-globe eye injuries
Bradycardia	Especially with repeated doses; vagotonic effect
Suxamethonium Apnoea	Due to deficiency or atypical forms of plasma cholinesterase
Myalgia	Due to initial fasciculations
Raised Intragastric Pressure	May increase aspiration risk (controversial)
Anaphylaxis	One of the most common agents associated with perioperative anaphylaxis

Pharmacokinetics

Suxamethonium is typically administered intravenously, though intramuscular administration is possible when IV access is not available. The onset of action is extremely rapid—within 45 s—and its duration is short, lasting approximately 7–10 min. It is rapidly hydrolysed by plasma cholinesterase, not acetylcholinesterase (Cook 2023). Structurally, it is composed of two acetylcholine molecules joined together. Pharmacokinetic studies confirm its very short distribution half-life and rapid plasma clearance (Torda et al. 1997) (Table 10.14).

Succinylcholine Apnoea

A rare but significant complication is prolonged apnoea in patients with atypical or deficient plasma cholinesterase. These individuals are unable to rapidly metabolise suxamethonium, resulting in extended paralysis that may last several hours (Norris 2003). Causes may be inherited (autosomal recessive trait) or acquired, including liver failure, pregnancy, burns, renal failure, malignancy, malnutrition, or exposure to certain drugs (e.g. esmolol, cyclophosphamide). Diagnosis is confirmed using the dibucaine number test, with normal values >70 (Trujillo 2023).

Contraindications

Suxamethonium is contraindicated in several clinical scenarios due to the risk of life-threatening complications such as hyperkalaemia or malignant hyperthermia. These include:

- Known or suspected malignant hyperthermia susceptibility
- Neuromuscular disorders, such as motor neuron disease or muscular dystrophies
- Burns, crush injuries, or immobilisation >24–48 h (risk of upregulated extrajunctional ACh receptors and resultant hyperkalaemia)
- Pre-existing hyperkalaemia or conditions with risk of potassium release (e.g. rhabdomyolysis)
- Open globe injuries, due to increased intraocular pressure
- Plasma cholinesterase deficiency (congenital or acquired) (Muñoz-Martínez 2015) (Table 10.15)

Table 10.15 Comparison of neuromuscular blocking agents

Drug	Type	Duration	Metabolism	Reversal agent	Histamine release	Key side effects	Typical dose
Rocuronium	Non-depolarising	30–60 min	Hepatic + biliary excretion	Sugammadex	No	Bradycardia, prolonged paralysis	0.6–1.2 mg/kg IV
Atracurium	Non-depolarising	20–35 min	Hofmann elimination + esterases	Neostigmine	Yes	Flushing, hypotension due to histamine release	0.5 mg/kg IV
Cisatracurium	Non-depolarising	30–40 min	Hofmann elimination	Neostigmine	No	Minimal cardiovascular effects	0.1–0.2 mg/kg IV
Vecuronium	Non-depolarising	30–40 min	Hepatic metabolism, renal excretion	Neostigmine / Sugammadex	No	Accumulation in liver failure, prolonged blockade	0.1 mg/kg IV
Pancuronium	Non-depolarising	90–180 min	Renal	Neostigmine	No	Tachycardia, prolonged action	0.1 mg/kg IV
Mivacurium	Non-depolarising	15–20 min	Plasma cholinesterase	Neostigmine	Yes	Bronchospasm, flushing	0.15–0.25 mg/kg IV
Suxamethonium	Depolarising	7–10 min	Plasma cholinesterase	None (supportive care)	Rare	Malignant hyperthermia, hyperkalaemia, myalgia, bradycardia, increased IOP & ICP	1–2 mg/kg IV

10.4 Local Anaesthetics

Local anaesthetics (LAs) are cornerstone agents in anaesthesia and pain medicine. They work by causing reversible loss of sensation in a targeted area of the body while preserving consciousness. By blocking nerve conduction—particularly in sensory neurons—they enable a wide range of surgical and analgesic interventions across settings such as infiltration anaesthesia (e.g. minor procedures), peripheral nerve blocks (e.g. brachial plexus), neuraxial blocks (spinal, epidural), topical applications (e.g. eye, airway), and intravenous regional anaesthesia (IVRA or Bier's block).

Mechanism of Action

Local anaesthetics block voltage-gated sodium channels (particularly Nav1.7 and Nav1.8) on neuronal membranes, preventing sodium influx and halting depolarisation. This blocks the propagation of action potentials and disrupts nerve transmission (Fozzard et al. 2011). They act preferentially on small, myelinated fibres—particularly Type A-delta and unmyelinated C fibres—thereby targeting pain and temperature first. LAs exhibit a use-dependent (or frequency-dependent) block: they bind more readily to sodium channels in the open or inactivated state, making actively firing neurons more susceptible to blockade (Chevrier et al. 2004).

Chemical Structure

All local anaesthetics share a common structural motif comprising three parts:

- An aromatic ring, which confers lipid solubility,
- An intermediate linkage, which determines whether the agent is an amide or an ester,
- A tertiary amine, which provides water solubility and enables ionisation.

A helpful mnemonic: *"AmIdes have an 'I' in the prefix"*. For example, lidocaine and bupivacaine are amides, while procaine is an ester (Becker and Reed 2006) (Table 10.16).

Physicochemical Properties

The clinical profile of a local anaesthetic—onset, potency, and duration—is dictated by three key physicochemical properties. pKa influences the onset, as only the non-ionised form can penetrate neuronal membranes. Most LAs have a pKa between

Table 10.16 Classification of local anaesthetics

Class	Examples	Metabolism
Amides	Lidocaine, Bupivacaine, Ropivacaine, Prilocaine	Hepatic metabolism via CYP450 enzymes
Esters	Procaine, Chloroprocaine, Tetracaine, Cocaine	Hydrolysed by plasma pseudocholinesterase

7.6 and 9.0; agents with a lower pKa (closer to physiological pH), such as lidocaine, act faster. Lipid solubility determines potency, with highly lipid-soluble agents like bupivacaine being more potent than less lipophilic agents such as lidocaine. Protein binding correlates with duration, as drugs that bind extensively to plasma and tissue proteins—such as ropivacaine and bupivacaine—exhibit longer durations of action (Taylor et al. 2019).

Clinical Considerations

Differential blockade follows a predictable order of fibre sensitivity: sympathetic fibres (B fibres) are blocked first, followed by pain and temperature fibres (C and A-delta), then touch and pressure (A-beta), and finally motor fibres (A-alpha), which are the most resistant (Sonawane 2023).

Additives can modify the effect of local anaesthetics:

- Adrenaline produces vasoconstriction, prolonging duration, reducing systemic absorption, and intensifying the block.
- Sodium bicarbonate raises pH, increasing the proportion of non-ionised drug and speeding onset.
- Opioids, when added to neuraxial LAs, offer synergistic analgesia.
- Alpha-2 agonists like clonidine and dexmedetomidine prolong block duration.

Toxicity

The most serious complication is Local Anaesthetic Systemic Toxicity (LAST). Early signs involve the CNS—such as tinnitus, perioral numbness, agitation, and seizures—followed by cardiovascular toxicity including bradycardia, hypotension, ventricular arrhythmias, and cardiac arrest. Bupivacaine is notably cardiotoxic. Management includes 20% lipid emulsion therapy, airway protection, seizure control, and adherence to ACLS protocols (Mahajan 2022).

Choosing an Agent

Selection is guided by the desired onset, duration, safety profile, and intended application. Lidocaine is often used for rapid onset, bupivacaine for long-acting blocks, and ropivacaine for prolonged analgesia with reduced cardiotoxicity. Clinical context—such as spinal anaesthesia, wound infiltration, or continuous nerve block—determines the most appropriate agent.

10.4.1 Amide Local Anaesthetics

Amide local anaesthetics form the cornerstone of modern regional anaesthesia due to their favourable pharmacokinetics, chemical stability, and relatively low allergenic potential. Compared to ester local anaesthetics, amides are typically longer-acting and safer, making them widely used in a variety of clinical settings including infiltration, nerve blocks, neuraxial anaesthesia, and intravenous regional anaesthesia (Dillane and Finucane 2010).

Chemistry and Metabolism

Amide local anaesthetics are defined by the presence of an amide (-CONH-) bond between the aromatic ring and the amine group. This structural characteristic imparts greater chemical stability than their ester counterparts. Metabolism occurs primarily in the liver via cytochrome P450 enzymes—particularly CYP1A2 and CYP3A4 (Ekström and Gunnarsson 1996). As a result, these agents have longer half-lives and durations of action, but their use requires caution in patients with hepatic impairment, where drug accumulation may increase the risk of systemic toxicity (Dillane and Finucane 2010).

Common Amide Local Anaesthetics

Drugs in this class include lidocaine, bupivacaine, ropivacaine, levobupivacaine, mepivacaine, prilocaine, and etidocaine. A helpful mnemonic is: *"AmIdes have an 'I' in the prefix"*.

Individual Agents – Key Features

- **Lidocaine** is the gold standard for comparison among local anaesthetics. It has a rapid onset and intermediate duration of action, making it highly versatile. It is commonly used for infiltration, peripheral nerve blocks, spinal, and epidural anaesthesia. The maximum recommended dose is 3 mg/kg without adrenaline and 7 mg/kg with adrenaline (Dillane and Finucane 2010).
- **Bupivacaine** has a slower onset but offers a prolonged duration of anaesthesia. It provides excellent sensory block with relatively less motor block, making it well suited to neuraxial techniques. However, it is significantly cardiotoxic—particularly when administered as a bolus intravenously—and must be used with caution. The typical maximum dose is 2 mg/kg (Dillane and Finucane 2010).
- **Levobupivacaine**, the S-enantiomer of bupivacaine, provides similar efficacy with a better safety profile, particularly regarding cardiovascular toxicity. It is preferred in regional blocks and obstetric anaesthesia where haemodynamic stability is critical (Bardsley et al. 1998).
- **Ropivacaine** is structurally related to bupivacaine but has lower lipid solubility, resulting in reduced motor blockade and a lower risk of cardiotoxicity. These properties make it well suited for ambulatory surgery, obstetrics, and situations requiring prolonged sensory blockade with motor sparing (Ekström and Gunnarsson 1996).
- **Prilocaine** has an intermediate onset and duration of action and is less toxic than lidocaine. However, at high doses, it may induce methaemoglobinaemia due to the formation of o-toluidine metabolites. This effect is dose-dependent and more commonly observed in intravenous regional anaesthesia (IVRA) (Shibuya et al. 2021).
- **Mepivacaine** shares many similarities with lidocaine but has a slightly longer duration of action. However, it is not routinely used in obstetric anaesthesia due to concerns regarding higher foetal toxicity (Dillane and Finucane 2010).

- **Etidocaine** offers a long duration of action and a relatively rapid onset. Despite these advantages, it causes excessive motor blockade, which limits its usefulness in clinical practice today (Dillane and Finucane 2010) (Table 10.17).

10.4.2 Ester Local Anaesthetics

Ester local anaesthetics were the first synthetic agents developed for clinical anaesthesia. While they have largely been replaced by amide local anaesthetics in modern practice, esters still serve specific roles—particularly in topical and ophthalmic procedures. Compared to amides, esters are chemically less stable, have shorter half-lives, and are more likely to cause allergic reactions. These allergic reactions are primarily attributed to their metabolism into para-aminobenzoic acid (PABA), a known allergen (Eggleston and Lush 1996).

Chemistry and Metabolism

Ester local anaesthetics are characterised by an ester linkage (-COO-) between their aromatic ring and amine group. They are rapidly hydrolysed in plasma by pseudocholinesterase (also known as plasma cholinesterase or butyrylcholinesterase), a process that leads to a short duration of action and a reduced risk of systemic accumulation. Notably, metabolism of esters does not rely on hepatic pathways, making them useful in patients with liver dysfunction. However, the production of PABA during metabolism accounts for their higher allergenic potential compared to amide local anaesthetics (Eggleston and Lush 1996).

Common Ester Local Anaesthetics

- **Procaine (Novocaine):** Once widely used but now rarely employed due to its slow onset, short duration of action, and high potential for allergic reactions. Its clinical efficacy is considered poor in comparison with modern alternatives.
- **Chloroprocaine:** Has a very rapid onset and a short duration of action, making it ideal for obstetric anaesthesia when urgent surgical conversion (e.g. to caesarean section) is needed. It is considered relatively safe due to its rapid hydrolysis by plasma cholinesterase (Tonder et al. 2023).
- **Tetracaine (Amethocaine):** A highly potent and long-acting ester local anaesthetic. It is most commonly used in ophthalmology and for spinal anaesthesia. Due to its potency, it carries a higher risk of systemic toxicity and must be dosed carefully.
- **Benzocaine:** Poorly water soluble and used exclusively for topical anaesthesia, such as in lozenges, oral gels, and throat sprays. Its use has been associated with methaemoglobinaemia, particularly in children and when applied over large surface areas (Sewell and Rivey 2018).
- **Cocaine:** The only local anaesthetic with intrinsic vasoconstrictive properties due to inhibition of noradrenaline reuptake. It continues to be used in ENT and nasal procedures for both its anaesthetic and haemostatic effects. However, it has a high potential for abuse and causes central nervous system stimulation. Caution is warranted in patients with coronary artery disease, hypertension, or arrhythmias (Table 10.18).

Table 10.17 Amide local anaesthetics

Drug	Onset	Duration	Max dose (mg/kg)	Cardiotoxicity	Unique features	Common uses
Lidocaine	Fast	Intermediate (1–2 h)	3 (7 with adrenaline)	Low	Anti-arrhythmic; rapid onset	Infiltration, nerve block, IVRA
Bupivacaine	Moderate	Long (4–8 h)	2	High	Excellent sensory block; potent	Epidural, spinal, nerve block
Levobupivacaine	Moderate	Long (4–8 h)	2	Lower than bupivacaine	S-enantiomer; safer cardiac profile	Neuraxial and peripheral blocks
Ropivacaine	Moderate	Long (4–6 h)	3	Low	Less motor block; less lipid soluble	Obstetrics, ambulatory anaesthesia
Prilocaine	Moderate	Intermediate (2–4 h)	6	Low	Risk of methaemoglobinaemia at high doses	IVRA, dental, infiltration
Mepivacaine	Fast	Intermediate (2–3 h)	4	Moderate	Not recommended in obstetrics	Regional blocks, infiltration
Etidocaine	Fast	Long (5–10 h)	3	Moderate	Excessive motor block	Obsolete in most settings

Table 10.18 Ester local anaesthetics

Drug	Onset	Duration	Metabolism	Toxicity	Key features	Common uses
Procaine	Slow	Short (30–60 min)	Plasma cholinesterase	Low systemic; high allergy	Historical; poor efficacy	Rarely used
Chloroprocaine	Fast	Very short (20–30 min)	Plasma cholinesterase	Very low	Rapid onset, low toxicity	Epidural for urgent caesarean
Tetracaine	Slow	Long (2–3 h)	Plasma cholinesterase	Moderate–high	Potent, used for long spinal anaesthesia	Spinal, ophthalmic
Benzocaine	Very slow	Variable	Plasma cholinesterase	Methaemoglobinaemia	Topical only; insoluble	Lozenges, gels, sprays
Cocaine	Moderate	Intermediate (1 h)	Hepatic & plasma cholinesterase	High (CNS, CVS)	Vasoconstrictor, sympathomimetic, addictive	ENT and nasal surgery

Conflicts of Interest The authors have no conflicts of interest to declare that are relevant to the content of this chapter.

References

Adeyinka, A. and Senba, E., 2024. Neuromuscular blocking agents. In: *StatPearls* [Internet]. Treasure Island (FL): StatPearls Publishing. Available at: https://www.ncbi.nlm.nih.gov/books/NBK537168/

Alkire, M.T., Gorski, L.A. and Price, J.L., 2004. Relative amnesic potency of five inhalational anesthetics follows the Meyer–Overton rule. *Anesthesiology*, 101(2), pp.417–429. https://doi.org/10.1097/00000542-200408000-00022

Bardsley, H., Gristwood, R., Baker, H., Watson, N. and Nimmo, W.S., 1998. A comparison of the cardiovascular effects of levobupivacaine and rac-bupivacaine in healthy volunteers. *British Journal of Clinical Pharmacology*, 46(3), pp.245–249. https://doi.org/10.1046/j.1365-2125.1998.00074.x

Becker, D.E. and Reed, K.L., 2006. Essentials of local anesthetic pharmacology. *Anesthesia Progress*, 53(3), pp.98–109. https://doi.org/10.2344/0003-3006(2006)53[98:EOLAP]2.0.CO;2

Borgeat, A. and Stirnemann, H.R., 1998. Antiemetic effect of propofol. *Der Anaesthesist*, 47(9), pp.918–924. https://doi.org/10.1007/s001010050643

Butterworth, J.F. and Mackey, D.C., 2022. Barbiturates. In: *StatPearls* [Internet]. Treasure Island (FL): StatPearls Publishing. Available at: https://www.ncbi.nlm.nih.gov/books/NBK532277/

Chevrier, P., Vijayaragavan, K. and Chahine, M., 2004. Differential modulation of Nav1.7 and Nav1.8 peripheral nerve sodium channels by lidocaine and mexiletine. *British Journal of Pharmacology*, 142(3), pp.576–584. https://doi.org/10.1038/sj.bjp.0705812

Cook, T.M., 2023. Neuromuscular blockade. In: *StatPearls* [Internet]. Treasure Island (FL): StatPearls Publishing. Available at: https://www.ncbi.nlm.nih.gov/books/NBK538301/

Dhanasekaran, R., Owen, H. and Fraser, J.F., 2011. Halothane hepatitis: still a lingering problem. *Anaesthesia and Intensive Care*, 39(3), pp.414–421. PMID: 21675048

Dillane, D. and Finucane, B.T., 2010. Local anaesthetics: pharmacology and toxicity. *Canadian Journal of Anesthesia/Journal canadien d'anesthésie*, 57(11), pp.1043–1053. https://doi.org/10.1007/s12630-010-9338-9

Dinis-Oliveira, R.J., 2018. Metabolic profiles of propofol and fospropofol: clinical and forensic interpretative aspects. *BioMed Research International*, 2018, 6852857. https://doi.org/10.1155/2018/6852857

Doenicke, A., Soukup, J., Hoernecke, R. and Moss, J., 1997. The lack of histamine release with cisatracurium: a double-blind comparison with vecuronium. *Anesthesia & Analgesia*, 84(3), pp.623–628. https://doi.org/10.1097/00000539-199703000-00030

Driver, B.E., Klein, L.R., Schick, A.L., Levy, B., Miner, J.R. and Reardon, R.F., 2022. Recall of awareness during emergency department intubation: a prospective study. *Chest*, 162(4), pp.902–909. https://doi.org/10.1016/j.chest.2022.03.030

Dundee, J.W., 1984. Fifty years of thiopentone. *British Journal of Anaesthesia*, 56(3), pp.211–213. https://doi.org/10.1093/bja/56.3.211

Eggleston, S.T. and Lush, L.W., 1996. Understanding allergic reactions to local anesthetics. *Annals of Pharmacotherapy*, 30(7–8), pp.851–857. https://doi.org/10.1177/106002809603000724

Ekström, G. and Gunnarsson, U.B., 1996. Ropivacaine: a new amide-type local anesthetic agent, metabolized by cytochromes P450 1A2 and 3A4 in human liver microsomes. *Drug Metabolism and Disposition*, 24(9), pp.955–961. PMID: 8876938

Esper, T., Wehner, M., Meineke, H., Rueffert, H. and Bein, B., 2015. Blood/gas partition coefficients of volatile anaesthetics in a clinically relevant patient population. *British Journal of Anaesthesia*, 115(5), pp.764–769. https://doi.org/10.1093/bja/aev333

Flook, V., 1972. Safety aspects of the use of Entonox. *Anaesthesia*, 27(1), pp.43–51. https://doi.org/10.1111/j.1365-2044.1972.tb08155.x

Forman, S.A., 2011. Clinical and molecular pharmacology of etomidate. *Anesthesiology*, 114(3), pp.695–707. https://doi.org/10.1097/ALN.0b013e3181f2364b

Fozzard, H.A., Sheets, M.F. and Hanck, D.A., 2011. The sodium channel as a target for local anesthetic drugs. *Frontiers in Pharmacology*, 2, 68. https://doi.org/10.3389/fphar.2011.00068

Franks, N.P., 2006. Molecular targets underlying general anaesthesia. *British Journal of Pharmacology*, 147(S1), pp.S72–S81. https://doi.org/10.1038/sj.bjp.0706441

Frasca, V., Riazzi, B.S. and Matthews, R.G., 1986. In vitro inactivation of methionine synthase by nitrous oxide. *Journal of Biological Chemistry*, 261(34), pp.15823–15826. PMID: 3536916

Frink, E.J., Malan, T.P., Morgan, S.E., Brown, E.A., Malcomson, M. and Brown, B.R., 1992. Quantification of the degradation products of sevoflurane in two CO_2 absorbents during low-flow anesthesia in surgical patients. *Anesthesiology*, 77(6), pp.1064–1069. https://doi.org/10.1097/00000542-199212000-00009

Garcia, P.S., Kolesky, S.E. and Jenkins, A., 2010. General anesthetic actions on GABAAA receptors. *Cellular and Molecular Life Sciences*, 67(3), pp.362–376. https://doi.org/10.1007/s00018-009-0161-1

Govindarajan, R., Narayanan, J.T., Singh, P. and Gupta, M., 2004. Role of thiopentone infusion for management of intractable status epilepticus not responding to conventional pharmacotherapy. *Annals of Indian Academy of Neurology*, 7(1), pp.37–41. PMID: 21887164

Hager, H.H., Patel, P. and Burns, B., 2025. Succinylcholine chloride. In: *StatPearls* [Internet]. Treasure Island (FL): StatPearls Publishing. Available at: https://www.ncbi.nlm.nih.gov/books/NBK499984/

Hildreth, A.N., Mejia, V.A., Maxwell, R.A., Smith, P.W., Dart, B.W. and Barker, D.E., 2008. Adrenal suppression following a single dose of etomidate for rapid sequence induction: a prospective randomized study. *Journal of Trauma*, 65(3), pp.573–579. https://doi.org/10.1097/TA.0b013e31818255e8

Knuf, K.M. and Maani, C.V., 2025. Nitrous oxide. In: *StatPearls* [Internet]. Treasure Island (FL): StatPearls Publishing. Available at: https://www.ncbi.nlm.nih.gov/books/NBK537013/

Kurdi, M.S., Theerth, K.A. and Deva, R.S., 2014. Ketamine: current applications in anesthesia, pain, and critical care. *Anesthesia: Essays and Researches*, 8(3), pp.283–290. https://doi.org/10.4103/0259-1162.143110

Mahajan, A., 2022. Local anesthetic systemic toxicity. In: *StatPearls* [Internet]. Treasure Island (FL): StatPearls Publishing. Available at: https://www.ncbi.nlm.nih.gov/books/NBK499964/

Matta, B.F., Lam, A.M., Mayberg, T.S. and Eng, C.C., 1995. Cerebrovascular response to intravenous thiopental: effect of dose and role of sympathetic activity. *Anesthesiology*, 82(1), pp.123–133. https://doi.org/10.1097/00000542-199501000-00016

Mion, G., 2017. History of anaesthesia: the ketamine story – past, present and future. *European Journal of Anaesthesiology*, 34(9), pp.571–575. https://doi.org/10.1097/EJA.0000000000000633

Morris, C., Perris, A., Klein, J. and Mahoney, P., 2009. Anaesthesia in haemodynamically compromised emergency patients: does ketamine represent the best choice of induction agent? *Anaesthesia*, 64(5), pp.532–539. https://doi.org/10.1111/j.1365-2044.2008.05835.x

Moss, A.P., Al-Ghamdi, A., El-Beheiry, H., Pullockaran, A.D., Lukasik, V., Grosse, P., Kompanje, E.J., Orchard, M., Higgins, B., Zhou, N. and Erb, J.R., 2022. Sugammadex versus neostigmine for routine reversal of neuromuscular blockade: a meta-analysis. *Journal of Clinical Medicine*, 11(17), 5095. https://doi.org/10.3390/jcm11175095

Muñoz-Martínez, T., 2015. Contraindications to succinylcholine in the intensive care unit. *Anesthesia & Analgesia*, 120(1), pp.e7–e8. https://doi.org/10.1213/ANE.0000000000000450

Norris, J.C., 2003. Prolonged suxamethonium apnoea resulting from acquired deficiency of plasma cholinesterase. *Anaesthesia*, 58(11), pp.1137–1139. https://doi.org/10.1046/j.1365-2044.2003.03503.x

Parviainen, I., Kälviäinen, R. and Ruokonen, E., 2007. Propofol and barbiturates for the anesthesia of refractory convulsive status epilepticus: pros and cons. *Neurological Research*, 29(7), pp.667–671. https://doi.org/10.1179/016164107X240044

Peltoniemi, M.A., Hagelberg, N.M., Olkkola, K.T. and Saari, T.I., 2016. Ketamine: a review of clinical pharmacokinetics and pharmacodynamics in anesthesia and pain therapy. *Clinical Pharmacokinetics*, 55(9), pp.1059–1077. https://doi.org/10.1007/s40262-016-0383-6

Rampil, I.J., 1994. Anesthetic potency is not altered after hypothermic spinal cord transection in rats. *Anesthesiology*, 80(4), pp.606–610. https://doi.org/10.1097/00000542-199404000-00003

Renou, A.M., D'Athis, P., Ecoffey, C., Guesde, R. and Ferec, C., 1978. Cerebral blood flow and metabolism during etomidate anaesthesia. *Anesthesiology*, 48(2), pp.111–117. https://doi.org/10.1097/00000542-197802000-00005

Ritz, M.L., 2023. Atracurium. In: *StatPearls* [Internet]. Treasure Island (FL): StatPearls Publishing. Available at: https://www.ncbi.nlm.nih.gov/books/NBK499995/

Sahinovic, M.M., Struys, M.M.R.F. and Absalom, A.R., 2018. Clinical pharmacokinetics and pharmacodynamics of propofol. *Clinical Pharmacokinetics*, 57(12), pp.1543–1568. https://doi.org/10.1007/s40262-018-0672-3

Sener, S., Eken, C., Schultz, C.H., Serinken, M. and Ozsarac, M., 2011. Ketamine with and without midazolam for emergency department sedation in adults: a randomized controlled trial. *Annals of Emergency Medicine*, 57(2), pp.109–114.e2. https://doi.org/10.1016/j.annemergmed.2010.09.010

Shahani, R., Streutker, C., Dickson, B. and Stewart, R.J., 2007. Ketamine-associated ulcerative cystitis: a new clinical entity. *Urology*, 69(5), pp.810–812. https://doi.org/10.1016/j.urology.2007.01.038

Shibata, Y., Kojima, T., Aoki, M., Hirosawa, S. and Iwasaka, H., 2016. Injury due to extravasation of thiopental and propofol. *Anesthesia & Analgesia*, 122(1), pp.54–60. https://doi.org/10.1213/ANE.0000000000001105

Shibuya, M., Nomura, T. and Guan, L., 2021. Methemoglobinemia caused by a low dose of prilocaine in a patient with renal failure. *Case Reports in Anesthesiology*, 2021, 5567532. https://doi.org/10.1155/2021/5567532

Shukla, A., Agarwal, K., Verma, N. and Gupta, D., 2010. Intraoperative bronchospasm with thiopental. *Indian Journal of Anaesthesia*, 54(6), pp.563–565. https://doi.org/10.4103/0019-5049.72670

Sewell, C.R. and Rivey, M.P., 2018. A case report of benzocaine-induced methemoglobinemia. *Journal of Pharmacy Practice*, 31(5), pp.507–509. https://doi.org/10.1177/0897190017723211

Sonawane, K., 2023. Nerve anatomy and physiology. In: *StatPearls* [Internet]. Treasure Island (FL): StatPearls Publishing. Available at: https://www.ncbi.nlm.nih.gov/books/NBK538331/

Taylor, A., McLeod, G. and Tunstall, M., 2019. Basic pharmacology of local anaesthetics. *BJA Education*, 19(11), pp.363–369. https://doi.org/10.1016/j.bjae.2019.07.001

Tonder, S., Togioka, B.M. and Maani, C.V., 2023. Chloroprocaine. In: *StatPearls* [Internet]. Treasure Island (FL): StatPearls Publishing. Available at: https://www.ncbi.nlm.nih.gov/books/NBK538331/

Torda, T.A., Graham, G.G., Warwick, N.R. and Donohue, P., 1997. Pharmacokinetics and pharmacodynamics of suxamethonium. *Anaesthesia and Intensive Care*, 25(3), pp.272–278. https://doi.org/10.1177/0310057X9702500312

Trujillo, R., 2023. Pseudocholinesterase deficiency. In: *StatPearls* [Internet]. Treasure Island (FL): StatPearls Publishing. Available at: https://www.ncbi.nlm.nih.gov/books/NBK541032/

Valk, B.I. and Struys, M.M.R.F., 2021. Etomidate and its analogs: a review of pharmacokinetics and pharmacodynamics. *Clinical Pharmacokinetics*, 60(10), pp.1253–1269. https://doi.org/10.1007/s40262-021-01038-6

Vasile, B., Rasulo, F., Candiani, A. and Latronico, N., 2003. The pathophysiology of propofol infusion syndrome: a simple name for a complex syndrome. *Intensive Care Medicine*, 29(9), pp.1417–1425. https://doi.org/10.1007/s00134-003-1850-6

Vinclair, M., Broux, C., Faure, P., Brun. J., Genty, C., Jacquot, C., Chabre, O., and Payen J-F., 2008. Duration of adrenal inhibition following a single dose of etomidate in critically ill patients. *Intensive Care Medicine*, 34(4), pp. 714–719. https://doi.org/10.1007/s00134-007-0970-y.

Questions on Pharmacology Fundamentals 11

Pharmacokinetics

What routes can be used to administer drugs
Define pharmacokinetics.
What are first order kinetics?
What are zero order kinetics?
What are Michaelis-Menton kinetics?
What factors influence drug absorption?
What is pKa?
How does pKa influence drug absorption?
What is the Henderson-Hasselbalch equation?
How is the Henderson-Hasselbach equation used to predict drug absorption
Define bioavailability?
How is bioavailability measured?
What factors influence bioavailability?
What is first pass metabolism
Give examples of first pass metabolism?
What is the hepatic extraction ratio?
What routes of administration avoid first pass metabolism?
What factors influence transdermal absorption?
List some disadvantages of intramuscular drug administration.
What effect does particle size have on inhalational drug administration?
What is a pro-drug?
How can drugs be metabolised?
Discuss the difference between elimination and excretion.
List the main sites of drug excretion.
Discuss the considerations of drug administration in renal disease.
What is the compartment model of drug administration?
Describe the 1-compartment model.

G. Browne, *PharmacologyPro*, https://doi.org/10.1007/978-3-032-10227-0_11

Describe the 2-compartment model.
How is 2-compartment model different from a 3-compartment model?
What is context sensitive half-life?
What causes context sensitive half-life?
What is context insensitive half-life?
What is Volume of Distribution?
List some factors which affect the Volume of Distribution
How is volume of distribution calculated in a One Compartment Model?
What is Half-Life?
What is Clearance?
How could you calculate the rate of elimination?
What is the elimination half-life?
How are volume of distribution, clearance and half-life interrelated?
What is a time constant?
Compare and contrast time contrast and half-life.
Why can some drugs be given as repeated dose and some need infusion?
How do lipophilicity and hydrophilicity affect drug distribution?
Why do some drugs accumulate in fat or bone?
How does protein binding affect drug distribution and elimination?
What clinical relevance does high protein binding have?
What is the difference between free and total drug concentration?
How does hypoalbuminaemia affect drug dosing?
Why are loading doses used and how are they calculated?
Why do elderly patients often require lower drug doses?
How does obesity affect volume of distribution and clearance?
What is the difference between peak and trough drug levels?
What is steady state and how is it achieved?
How many half-lives does it take to reach steady state?
Why are maintenance doses important?
What is meant by clearance being 'flow limited' versus 'capacity limited'?
How does hepatic blood flow affect drug clearance?
How can renal function be assessed when adjusting doses?
What is creatinine clearance and how is it estimated?
What drugs require therapeutic drug monitoring?
Give examples of drugs with narrow therapeutic windows.
What is non-linear pharmacokinetics and give examples?
How does saturation of enzymes affect drug kinetics?
What is the significance of redistribution in IV anaesthetic drugs?
How is drug accumulation assessed?

Pharmacodynamics

Define Pharmacodynamics
How do drugs exert their effects?
What is an enzyme?

What is a ligand?
What is a receptor?
What governs drug-receptor interactions?
Do all ligands initiate a response on binding to receptor?
How do you classify receptors?
What are the main mechanisms of receptor action?
What do you know about the G-Protein Coupled Receptor?
What is the structure of the G-Protein Coupled Receptor?
What happens when a GPCR is activated?
What are G-proteins?
What are the main types of G-proteins?
Give examples of G-protein interactions.
How do phosphodiesterase inhibitors work?
What do you know about the insulin receptor?
Give examples of physicochemical properties of drugs.
Give examples of drugs interacting with enzymes.
Give examples of drugs altering ion permeability.
Give examples of drugs exerting it's effect by reducing ion permeability.
Give examples of intermediate messenger and ligands activating them.
What are second messengers and name examples?
How do nuclear receptors differ from membrane-bound receptors?
How do ion channel receptors function?
What are tyrosine kinase receptors?
How is receptor upregulation and downregulation relevant clinically?
What is receptor reserve (spare receptors)?
What is the role of intracellular signalling cascades?
How do drugs differ in their speed of onset depending on receptor type?
What determines the selectivity of a drug?
What is the therapeutic index?
What is meant by receptor sensitivity?
Give an example of a drug that shows tolerance with repeated use.
What is the difference between desensitisation and receptor internalisation?
What is the difference between pharmacodynamic and pharmacokinetic tolerance?

Drug Interactions

What are drug interactions?
Classify drug interactions and give examples.
Tell me about cytochrome P450 system.
List some enzyme inducers.
List some enzyme inhibitors.
What is summation?
What is synergism?
What is potentiation?

What is the difference between pharmacokinetic and pharmacodynamic drug interactions?
Give examples of beneficial drug interactions in anaesthesia.
How do antacids affect drug absorption?
How do antibiotics affect the efficacy of oral contraceptives?
Give examples of life-threatening drug-drug interactions.
How does protein binding displacement affect drug action?
Why should SSRIs not be combined with MAO inhibitors?
What is serotonin syndrome?
How do fruit juices like grapefruit affect drug metabolism?
How do you manage polypharmacy in elderly patients?

Metabolism & Excretion

How are drugs metabolised by the liver?
What drugs cause damage to the liver?
How does chronic liver disease affect drug metabolism?
How are drugs excreted from the body?
Describe how drugs are handled as they pass through the kidney.
What are the effects of age on renal drug metabolism?
What is Phase I metabolism? Give examples.
What is Phase II metabolism? Give examples.
What enzymes are involved in Phase I reactions?
What is the role of conjugation in metabolism?
What is enterohepatic circulation?
How does pH of urine affect renal drug excretion?
How can forced diuresis alter drug excretion?
What is the impact of acidifying vs alkalinising the urine?
Give examples of drugs excreted unchanged by the kidneys.
Why do water-soluble drugs get cleared faster than lipid-soluble ones?

Variations in Drug Metabolism

Explain how genetic polymorphism influences drug metabolism
What clinical effects can genetic polymorphism have?
How would you manage someone with unexpected suxamethonium apnoea?
How is the enzyme abnormality diagnosed?
What other drugs are affected by genetic polymorphism?
What are poor, intermediate, extensive, and ultra-rapid metabolisers?
What enzyme variants affect codeine metabolism?
What is malignant hyperthermia and what mutation is associated?
What is G6PD deficiency and why is it relevant to pharmacology?
How does ethnicity influence drug metabolism patterns?
What pharmacogenomic tests are available clinically?

Why is thiopurine methyltransferase (TPMT) testing recommended before azathioprine?
What is the role of NAT2 polymorphism in drug metabolism?

Agonist and Antagonists
Define Affinity.
What is Intrinsic activity?
Define Potency.
How can you compare potency of drugs?
Define Efficacy.
What is EC50 and ED50?
Define Full Agonist.
Define Inverse agonist.
What is an Antagonist
Give examples of an antagonist.
What is an Allosteric modulator?
Compare and contrast tachyphylaxis and desensitisation?
What is the difference between competitive antagonist and an inverse agonist?
What is the dose-response curve and graph?
Describe log dose response curve.
How would the curve for a low potency drug compare to drug with a higher potency?
What moves the curve to the right?
What would happen the shape of the curve with a non-competitive antagonist?
What would happen if a partial agonist was given?
What is the dose ratio?
How does receptor affinity influence dose-response?
What is the clinical implication of a partial agonist?
How do irreversible antagonists work?
How can antagonism be overcome?
What is functional antagonism?
What is chemical antagonism?
Describe examples of non-receptor antagonism.
What is receptor desensitisation and how does it develop?
What is meant by ceiling effect in partial agonists?
Explain spare receptors using an example.
How do you interpret a Schild plot?
What happens to efficacy in presence of competitive vs non-competitive antagonists?

Isomerism
What are isomers?
Classify the different types of isomers.
What are structural isomers? Give an example.

What is tautomerism? Give an example.
What are stereoisomers? Give an example.
What is a chiral centre? Give an example of a drug with a chiral centre.
What is a racemic mixture?
What is an enantiopure preparation?
Do physiological enantiomers exist?
What is the clinical relevance of isomerism?
Why might one enantiomer be more potent or less toxic than its mirror image?
Give an example of a racemic mixture in anaesthesia.
How do enantiomers differ in metabolism or receptor binding?
What is optical isomerism?
What is geometric isomerism?
What is the relevance of isomerism in local anaesthetics?
Why was levobupivacaine developed?
What is stereoselective metabolism?
How can isomerism affect pharmacodynamics?
How do regulatory authorities treat racemic versus single-enantiomer drugs?

Questions on Clinical Drugs

12

Anti-Arrhythmic Drugs
Classify antiarrhythmics.
Tell me about Vaughn-Williams classification and give examples.
How do class I drugs exert their effects?
How do class II drugs exert their effects?
How do class III drugs exert their effects?
How do class IV drugs exert their effects?
What are the limitations of the Vaughn-Williams classification?
Tell me more about classification of anti-arrhythmic according to clinical use
What drugs used for supra-ventricular arrhythmias?
What is Adenosine used for?
What is the mechanism of action of Adenosine?
What is Verapamil used for?
What is the mechanism of action of Verapamil?
Discuss the main difference between verapamil and nifedipine?
What drugs can be used to treat Atrial Fibrillation?
What are the clinical uses of digoxin?
What is the mechanism of action of digoxin?
What are the symptoms and signs of digoxin toxicity?
Discuss the treatment of digoxin toxicity.
What can amiodarone be used for?
How does amiodarone work?
List the side effects of amiodarone.
Why is amiodarone effective in both atrial and ventricular arrhythmias?
What are the pharmacokinetics of amiodarone and how do they impact dosing?
How does dronedarone compare to amiodarone?
What precautions are needed before administering adenosine?
Why is verapamil contraindicated with beta blockers?
What are the ECG changes associated with digoxin toxicity?

G. Browne, *PharmacologyPro*, https://doi.org/10.1007/978-3-032-10227-0_12

How is sotalol classified and what are its dual effects?
Why is lidocaine preferred in ischaemic ventricular arrhythmias?
What role does magnesium play in arrhythmia management?

Anti-Hypertensive Agents
Classify antihypertensives.
What do you know about beta blockers?
Discuss their uses and side effects.
What anti-hypertensives are used to treat hypertensive emergencies?
Tell me about sodium nitroprusside.
Discuss Cyanide toxicity, it's presentation and treatment.
What is a diuretic?
Classify diuretics.
How does each class work?
Draw a nephron and indicate where diuretics exert their effects.
How does mannitol exert its effect?
What are the main indication for mannitol?
Can mannitol be used repeatedly?
What are the main indication for diuretics?
Discuss the side effects of thiazides.
What are the side effects of loop diuretics?
How are diuretics used in renal failure?
Briefly explain the RAAS system.
What are the common side effects of anti-hypertensive agents?
What are the anaesthetic implications of chronic ACE inhibitor use?
Why can beta blockers cause bradycardia and bronchospasm?
What is the mechanism of action of hydralazine?
How does clonidine reduce blood pressure and how is it used in anaesthesia?
What are the central vs peripheral alpha-blockers?
Why is labetalol preferred in pregnancy-induced hypertension?
How do potassium-sparing diuretics work and when are they used?
What is rebound hypertension and which drugs cause it?

Inotropes & Vasopressors
What is an inotrope?
What is a vasopressor?
Name some positively inotropic drugs.
How does digoxin act as an inotrope?
When do you give calcium and why is it important in cardiac contractility?
How does dobutamine work?
Compare and contrast ephedrine and phenylephrine.
Give some uses for adrenaline.
What is the mechanism of action of adrenaline?

Discuss the side effects of adrenaline.
Compare and contrast adrenaline and noradrenaline.
How are adrenaline and noradrenaline metabolised?
What are the anaesthetic implications of using high-dose vasopressors?
How does vasopressin exert its effects and when is it used?
Compare the use of dobutamine vs milrinone in low cardiac output states.
What is the effect of pH and acidosis on vasopressor efficacy?
What is the mechanism of action of levosimendan?
Why is noradrenaline the vasopressor of choice in septic shock?

Analgesics
What is the difference between an opiate and an opioid?
Classify opioid receptors
What is the action and distribution of each opioid receptor?
How do opioids work at a molecular level?
What routes of administration can opioids be used with?
What are the unwanted side effects of opioids?
What is tolerance?
What is dependence?
What is addiction?
Describe the symptoms of opioid withdrawal.
Discuss the pharmacodynamic effects of opioids.
Why do fentanyl, morphine and alfentanil have different onset times?
How is morphine metabolised and excreted?
Tell me about remifentanil.
What is the mode of action of NSAIDS?
Describe the action of cyclooxygenases.
What are the actions of prostaglandin and prostacyclin?
Classify NSAIDS.
What are the uses for NSAIDS?
What are the main side effects of NSAIDS?
Difference between COX-1 and COX-2 inhibition
What are the respective side effects of COX-1 and COX-2?
Compare and contrast diclofenac and ibuprofen
How does paracetamol work?
How does paracetamol toxicity occur?
Why do opioids cause bradycardia and hypotension?
What is the difference in metabolism between fentanyl and morphine?
How does opioid-induced hyperalgesia occur?
Why does remifentanil require post-operative analgesia planning?
What is the ceiling effect in opioids?
What is the significance of CYP2D6 polymorphisms in codeine metabolism?
How is naloxone used in opioid toxicity?
Why is paracetamol considered safe in most patients?

Anticonvulsants
What is epilepsy and how is it classified?
List the drugs available to treat epilepsy
How do anti-epileptics work?
Describe the GABA receptor.
What is the mechanism of action of Phenytoin?
What is the mechanism of action of Sodium valproate?
What are the effects of anticonvulsants in pregnancy?
Describe the management of status epilepticus.
What is gabapentin commonly used for?
Can propofol be used in epilepsy?
What are the interactions of anti-epileptic drugs with anaesthetic agents?
Why is sodium valproate avoided in young women?
What is the anaesthetic consideration for a patient on long-term carbamazepine?
What is the difference between focal and generalised seizure pharmacotherapy?

Antidepressants
What are the different classes of antidepressant agents?
Describe the mode of action of the different classes of antidepressants
What are the side effects of antidepressants?
What is serotonin syndrome?
What are the perioperative considerations of SSRIs?
Why are tricyclic antidepressants dangerous in overdose?
What are the risks of combining MAOIs with anaesthesia?
What precautions are taken with patients on chronic antidepressants?

Benzodiazepines
What are benzodiazepines?
Describe the effects of benzodiazepines.
What is the mechanism of action of benzodiazepines?
How are benzodiazepines metabolised?
What are the advantages of midazolam pre-operatively?
Discuss the treatment of benzodiazepine overdose and antidote.
What is the mechanism and half-life of flumazenil?
Why is flumazenil contraindicated in chronic benzodiazepine users?
What is the risk of re-sedation after flumazenil?
How does tolerance to benzodiazepines develop?

Drugs Acting on the GI Tract
Classify drugs acting on the GIT
How is gastric acid produced?
What increases gastric acid secretion?

What do we use to reduce gastric acid secretion?
What is the role of prostaglandin in gastric acid secretion?
Do we use prostaglandin analogues? Give examples.
What drugs do we use to protect gastric mucosa?
What do you mean by pro-kinetics? Give examples and mechanism of action.
How does ranitidine differ from omeprazole in mechanism and use?
What is the role of erythromycin in gastric motility?
Why is metoclopramide contraindicated in Parkinson's disease?
What is the serotonin receptor's role in emetogenesis?
How does dexamethasone exert antiemetic effects?

Anti-Emetics
Discuss the physiology of vomiting.
How is vomiting controlled?
Summarise the receptors involved in initiating vomiting
What are the locations of the receptors involved in vomiting?
Classify anti-emetics.
What is the mechanism of action of Ondansetron?
Discuss the side effects of Ondansetron
What is the mechanism of action of Cyclizine?
Discuss the side effects of Cyclizine
What is the mechanism of action of Metoclopramide?
Discuss the side effects of Metoclopramide
What are the features of neuroleptic malignant syndrome?
Discuss the treatment of neuroleptic malignant syndrome.
What antiemetics can be used safely in Parkinson's Disease?
What are NK1 receptors?
What can you do to reduce the incidence of Post-Operative N+V?
Which drugs increase gastric motility? How do they exert their effects?
Which drugs inhibit gastric motility? How do they exert their effects?

Antidiabetic Medication
Define diabetes mellitus. How is it classified?
How is diabetes mellitus diagnosed?
What is the clinical relevance of impaired fasting glucose and impaired glucose tolerance?
What is the mechanism of action of insulin?
What are the side effects of insulin?
How are insulin agents classified?
What drugs can be used to reduce blood sugar in DM?
What classes of drugs to treat type 1 DM?
Discuss the different types of insulin regimes available to patients?
What classes of drugs can be used to treat type 2 DM?

Discuss sulphonylureas.
What is the mechanism of action and side effects of sulphonylureas?
Discuss biguanides.
What is the mechanism of action and side effects of metformin?
Discuss the short-term and long-term complications of diabetes.
Discuss diabetes mellitus and its implications in anaesthesia.
What are the signs of hypoglycaemia under general anaesthesia?
Why is metformin held preoperatively?
How does insulin requirement change during surgery?
What are the interactions of steroids with diabetic control?
What is DKA and how is it managed perioperatively?

Asthma Pharmacology
What is asthma? Describe its basic pathophysiology.
Describe the pathophysiology of severe and life-threatening asthma.
Discuss the symptoms and signs of severe asthma.
Outline the pharmacological steps in the management of asthma.
Discuss drug treatment of severe and life-threatening asthma.
Which drugs should be avoided in acute severe/life-threatening asthma?
How do beta-agonists work in asthma?
What are the side effects of beta-agonists?
What is the role of magnesium sulphate in asthma?
Why are inhaled steroids not used acutely?
What is the anaesthetic management of a known asthmatic?

Anticoagulants
What are anticoagulants?
How are anticoagulants classified?
What is the mechanism of action of heparin?
List some common uses of heparin.
What types of heparin do you know?
How is heparin administered and why is it administered in this way?
What are the advantages of low molecular heparins?
How is heparin therapy monitored?
What are the side effects of heparin?
What is Heparin-Induced Thrombocytopenia (HIT)?
How would you reverse heparin?
What is the mechanism of action of warfarin?
Discuss the side effects of warfarin.
List some of the drug interactions of warfarin.
What factors potentiate the effect of warfarin?
How is warfarin therapy monitored?
List the ways to reverse warfarin, including rough timings.

What other anticoagulants do you know?
How can these anticoagulants be reversed?
What are the newer oral anticoagulants (DOACs) and how do they work?
How is bleeding managed in patients on DOACs?
When should aspirin or clopidogrel be withheld before surgery?
What are platelet function tests and how are they interpreted?
When are antifibrinolytics like tranexamic acid used?

Antiplatelets
Classify anti platelet drugs.
What is the mechanism of action of the different classes?
How are platelets involved in clotting?
What are some of the common uses of anti-platelet drugs, clinically?
Discuss the peri-operative considerations for anti-platelet agents.
How do fibrinolytic agents work?
When are fibrinolytic drugs used?
What is thromboelastometry monitoring? What are the advantages?

Blood
Describe the composition of stored red cell concentrate.
Discuss the risks associated with transfusion.
Discuss the benefits associated with transfusion.
What constitutes a massive transfusion?
What problems are associated with a massive transfusion?
What blood conservation strategies are available?
How long do platelets last in storage?
What is fresh frozen plasma?
What are the indications for cryoprecipitate?
How is transfusion-related lung injury (TRALI) diagnosed?
What are the storage conditions for each blood component?
How is transfusion-induced hyperkalaemia managed?

Local Anaesthetics
What are the main classes of local anaesthetics?
Give an example from each class.
How do local anaesthetics exert their effect?
What is the significance of pKa on local anaesthetics?
What is the significance of lipid solubility?
What is the significance of protein binding?
What is local anaesthetic potency related to?
What factor governs duration of action?
What factor governs speed of onset?

What are the side effects of lidocaine and bupivacaine?
Why do local anaesthetics not work in infected tissue?
What is heavy Marcaine?
What are the maximum doses of commonly used local anaesthetics with and without adrenaline?
What are the symptoms and signs of local anaesthetic toxicity?
What factors pre-disposing to local anaesthetic toxicity?
Discuss the management of local anaesthetic toxicity.
What is EMLA?
How does the rate of systemic vascular absorption vary?
How does pH buffering enhance local anaesthetic onset?
Why is ropivacaine preferred over bupivacaine in certain blocks?
What is the role of adrenaline in local anaesthesia?
How does intravascular injection of LA manifest clinically?
What is the mechanism of lipid emulsion in LAST treatment?

Intravenous Anaesthetic Agents
Discuss the uses of propofol
What is the mechanism of action of propofol?
What are the pharmacokinetics and side effects of propofol?
What is Thiopentone?
What is the mechanism of action of Thiopentone?
Discuss the uses of Ketamine?
What is the mechanism of action of Ketamine?
What are the pharmacokinetics and side effects of Ketamine?
What is TIVA?
List some indications for TIVA.
What is meant by TCI?
Which drugs lend themselves well to infusion regimes?
What is unique about remifentanil infusion?
What are the antiemetic properties of propofol?
Why is ketamine useful in haemodynamically unstable patients?
What are the contraindications to ketamine?
What are the differences between etomidate and propofol?
What are the endocrine effects of etomidate?

Inhalational Anaesthetic Agents
What is an inhalation agent?
What are the properties of an ideal anaesthetic agent?
What properties determine the potency and the onset of action?
What is the significance of blood:gas partition coefficient?
What is the significance of the oil:gas partition coefficient?
Define MAC
What factors affect MAC?

What is compound A?
Are there any harmful effects of inhalational anaesthetic agents?
How do inhalational agents exert their effects?
What neurotransmitters are implicated in the mode of action of anaesthetic agents?
What is halothane hepatitis and what causes it?
What do you know about xenon and its potential use in anaesthesia?
What do you know about helium?
What are the uses of nitrous oxide?
How is nitrous oxide stored?
What are the pharmacodynamic properties of Nitrous Oxide?
What are the advantages and disadvantages of Nitrous Oxide?
What is Entonox?
Explain the Concentration Effect associated with Nitrous Oxide.
Explain the Second Gas Effect associated with Nitrous Oxide.
Explain Diffusion Hypoxia.
How do volatile agents affect cerebral blood flow and ICP?
What is the role of sevoflurane in paediatric induction?
Why is desflurane not used for induction?
What are the occupational exposure limits for inhaled agents?

Neuromuscular Blocking Agents and Anticholinesterases
What is the neuromuscular junction?
Draw the NMJ.
Describe the nicotinic acetylcholine receptor.
How is ACh synthesised and subsequently broken down?
Classify drugs producing neuromuscular blockade.
Tell me about depolarising neuromuscular blockade.
How do non-depolarising muscle relaxants work?
Classify non-depolarising muscle relaxants
How are non-depolarising muscle relaxants metabolised?
What factors affect the speed of onset?
What are ED50 and ED95?
Tell me about metabolism of atracurium?
What are the side effects of atracurium?
What is cis-atracurium?
Tell me about the different intubating doses of rocuronium.
How do antibiotics modify action of non-depolarising neuromuscular blockers?
What other drugs modify the action of non-depolarising neuromuscular blockers?
What are the properties of an ideal neuromuscular blocker?
What factors affect the speed of recovery from non-depolarising muscle relaxation?
What monitoring is used to assess neuromuscular blockade?
What is train-of-four and how is it interpreted?
What is post-tetanic count?
How do magnesium and lithium affect NMBAs?

Suxamethonium
What class of drug is suxamethonium?
Describe it's structure.
What is the mechanism of action?
What are the side effects of suxamethonium?
What are the contraindications of suxamethonium?
What is 'sux apnoea'? How does it occur?
Discuss the management of sux apnoea.
Why is sux contraindicated in burns and neuromuscular disease?
What electrolyte changes occur with sux?
What are fasciculations and how can they be reduced?

Malignant Hyperpyrexia
What is malignant hyperpyrexia?
What are the signs and symptoms?
How is it managed?
What is dantrolene and how does it work?
Discuss the pathophysiology of malignant hyperpyrexia.
How do you diagnose malignant hyperpyrexia in relatives?
What agents are contraindicated in susceptible patients?
How is MH risk assessed preoperatively?
What is the caffeine-halothane contracture test?

Anti-Cholinesterases and Anti-Muscarinics
Discuss the different types of acetylcholine (ACh) receptor.
How is ACh synthesised?
What happens to ACh after its synthesis?
Tell me about acetylcholinesterase inhibitors, what uses do they have?
How do anticholinesterases exert their effects?
What are the disadvantages of acetylcholinesterase inhibitors?
Classify the three types of acetylcholinesterase inhibitors.
How does neostigmine reverse neuromuscular block?
What are the side effects of a conventional dose of neostigmine?
How do organophosphates work? What is the treatment of poisoning?
How do anti-muscarinics work?
What are the clinical uses of anti-muscarinics?
Describe the structure of hyoscine, atropine and glycopyrrolate.
Compare and contrast hyoscine, glycopyrrolate and atropine.
What are the side effects of these agents?
What are the differences in central penetration between antimuscarinics?
How do antimuscarinics affect heart rate and secretions?
Why is glycopyrrolate often paired with neostigmine?

Sugammadex

What is Sugammadex?
What are the advantages of this drug?
Can it be used with other neuromuscular blocking agents?
What are the disadvantages of sugammadex?
Discuss the different doses for use in different clinical settings.
How does sugammadex differ from neostigmine mechanistically?
Can sugammadex reverse profound blockade?
What allergic reactions are associated with sugammadex?
What are its limitations in renal impairment?

Index

A

Absorption, 2, 9, 13, 14, 39, 72, 83, 115, 117, 118, 121, 123, 135, 138, 194, 203, 206, 216
Affinity, 3, 74, 166, 207
Agonist, 1–3, 5, 9, 34, 41, 42, 48–50, 52–54, 68, 69, 71, 72, 74, 75, 83, 106, 116, 120, 121, 123, 175, 194, 207, 214
Amiodarone, 7, 18, 23–27, 81, 86, 158, 209
Anaesthesia exams, 206, 214, 216, 217
Analgesics, 211
Antagonist, 1–3, 5, 80–82, 84, 85, 88, 92, 100, 107, 110, 137, 158, 163, 175, 207
Anti-arrhythmics, 23–25, 28, 30, 95, 209
Anticoagulants, 63, 102, 103, 134, 148, 152, 153, 155, 156, 158, 159, 161, 214, 215
Anticonvulsants, 91, 94, 95, 97, 108, 111, 174, 176, 177, 180, 181, 212
Antidepressants, 6, 40, 99, 101–105, 107, 212
Antiemetics, 79–88, 174, 176, 177, 213, 216
Antihypertensives, 10, 28, 29, 33, 41, 134
Antiplatelet, 63–66, 102, 146, 152, 159–168, 215

B

Benzodiazepines, 3, 5, 42, 70, 71, 91, 92, 108–111, 179, 184, 212
Beta-blockers, 6, 27, 29, 31–33, 47, 209, 210
Bioavailability, 14, 15, 25, 27, 29, 32, 35, 37, 39, 41, 42, 52, 65, 66, 70, 74, 75, 81–83, 85–88, 93–95, 97, 98, 101, 104, 106, 107, 117, 119–122, 125, 133, 134, 136, 138, 139, 150, 153–155, 157, 158, 162, 163, 165, 179, 203
Bupivacaine, 10, 193–195, 197, 216

C

Calcium channel blockers (CCBs), 24, 27, 31–34
Central nervous system (CNS) depression, 110, 176
Clearance, 6, 8, 16–18, 20, 93, 157, 165, 166, 191, 204
Clinical scenarios, 158, 162, 191
COX inhibition, *see* Cyclooxygenase (COX) inhibition
Cyclizine, 80, 84–86, 213
Cyclooxygenase (COX) inhibition, 160–162

D

Diabetes mellitus (DM), 115, 116, 213, 214
Diabetic ketoacidosis (DKA), 115, 126, 127, 214
Digoxin, 1, 2, 23–28, 32, 41, 209, 210
Direct oral anticoagulants (DOACs), 152, 158, 215
Distribution, 2, 14, 17–20, 25, 71, 73, 176, 191, 204, 211
Diuretics, 33, 41, 120, 131–134, 136, 137, 139, 210
Dopamine antagonists, 80
Drug mechanisms, 175

E

Efficacy, 2, 10, 23, 25, 39, 52, 74, 80, 83, 85, 96, 101, 102, 134, 139, 145, 148, 149, 151, 159, 160, 164, 195, 196, 198, 206, 207, 211
Electrolyte imbalance, 23, 131, 139
Exam revision, 209–219
Excretion, 2, 15, 16, 18, 29, 30, 35, 42, 71, 81, 85–88, 95, 97, 106, 111, 131, 133, 134, 136, 138, 150, 163, 176, 179, 182, 192, 203, 206

G. Browne, *PharmacologyPro*, https://doi.org/10.1007/978-3-032-10227-0

F
Fentanyl, 2, 3, 7–9, 17, 19, 20, 67, 69, 71–73, 99, 211
Fibrinolytics, 150, 215
First-pass metabolism, 14, 15, 29, 35, 45, 70, 74, 81, 104, 162
5-HT_3 receptor, 83, 85
Flumazenil, 110, 111, 212

G
Gamma-aminobutyric acid (GABA), 3–5, 91, 92, 98, 109–111, 175, 176, 180, 182, 183, 212

H
Half-life, 8, 17, 18, 26, 27, 29, 30, 32, 35, 37, 39, 41, 42, 44, 46, 49, 50, 52, 54, 55, 65, 66, 70, 71, 73–75, 82, 83, 85–88, 93, 94, 97, 98, 101, 103, 104, 106, 107, 111, 117, 119–123, 125, 132–136, 138, 139, 150, 153, 155–158, 162, 165–167, 175, 176, 179, 182, 191, 204, 212
Heparin-induced thrombocytopenia (HIT), 157
Heparins, 152, 155–157, 214
Hypertension, 31, 32, 34–36, 38, 40, 42, 43, 45, 49, 53, 69, 103, 131–133, 135–137, 139, 164, 179, 185, 196, 210
Hypoglycaemia, 117–119, 121–125, 127, 214

I
Inhalational agents, 183–185, 217
Inotropes, 47, 48, 51, 210
Insulin, 3–5, 115–128, 134, 205, 213, 214
Insulin regimens, 127
Interactive learning, 203–208

K
Ketamine, 2, 3, 5, 10, 173–175, 177–180, 184, 216
Key concepts review, 203–208

L
Local anaesthetics, 1, 42, 43, 48–49, 72, 193–199, 208, 215, 216
Loop diuretics, 131, 132, 210

M
Mannitol, 131, 135, 210
MAOIs, *see* Monoamine oxidase inhibitors
MCQ practice, 203–208
Metabolism, 2, 6–10, 15, 16, 18, 20, 26, 27, 32, 37, 41, 44, 52, 61, 73–76, 82, 83, 86–88, 94, 95, 97, 98, 103, 106, 107, 109, 117, 119, 120, 122, 125, 126, 133–136, 138, 153, 158, 159, 165, 176, 180, 181, 185, 188, 189, 192, 193, 196, 203, 206–208, 211, 217
Metformin, 116–118, 122, 124, 126, 214
Metoclopramide, 80, 81, 83–84, 213
Monoamine oxidase inhibitors (MAOIs), 51, 74, 99, 100, 103–106, 212
Morphine, 1–3, 14–16, 67–71, 73–76, 85, 211

N
Naloxone, 1, 3, 68, 211
Nephron, 120, 131, 135, 139, 210
Neuroleptic malignant syndrome (NMS), 82, 84, 94, 213
Neuromuscular blockers, 187, 188, 190, 217
NK1 receptors, 80, 213
Non-steroidal anti-inflammatory drugs (NSAIDs), 61–64, 66, 74, 75, 102, 103, 119, 158, 162

O
Ondansetron, 80, 85–86, 88
Opioid-induced hyperalgesia, 211
Opioids, 6, 42, 64, 67, 74, 79, 81, 99, 105, 109–111, 183, 184, 194, 211

P
Paracetamol, 2, 8, 9, 46, 61, 66, 67, 74, 75, 211
Perioperative management, 40, 92, 146, 152
Pharmacodynamics, 23, 126, 176, 178, 180, 182, 185, 204, 208
Pharmacokinetics, 6, 17–19, 25, 27, 29, 30, 32, 35, 37, 39, 41, 42, 44, 45, 49, 50, 52–55, 65, 66, 70, 71, 73–75, 81–84, 86–88, 93–98, 101, 103, 104, 106, 107, 109, 111, 117, 119–123, 125, 133–136, 138, 139, 149, 150, 153, 155–158, 162, 163, 165, 166, 176, 179, 181, 186, 191, 194, 203, 204, 209, 216
Pharmacology questions, 203–208
Phenytoin, 6–9, 24, 25, 91, 92, 94–96, 99, 212
Platelet function tests, 215

Postoperative nausea and vomiting (PONV), 79, 84–86, 88, 176, 186
Potassium-sparing diuretics, 132, 210
Potency, 2, 9, 69, 70, 72, 127, 164, 179, 183, 184, 186, 193, 196, 207, 215, 216
Propofol, 3, 5, 8, 9, 17, 19, 174–177, 180–182, 212, 216

R

Receptor sensitivity, 205
Receptors, 1–4, 7, 24, 33, 92, 116, 132, 144, 160, 176
Remifentanil, 69, 72, 73, 174, 211, 216
Renal failure, 17, 70, 133, 135, 177, 191, 210
Renin–angiotensin–aldosterone system (RAAS), 34, 38, 210
Reversal agents, 152, 159
Rocuronium, 188–190, 192, 217

S

Selective serotonin reuptake inhibitors (SSRIs), 74, 99–102, 105–108, 212
Signal transduction, 13
Sodium valproate, 91, 92, 98, 212
Sugammadex, 188–190, 192, 219
Sulphonylureas, 118–119, 121–124, 214
Suxamethonium, 16, 188–192, 218

T

Therapeutic index (TI), 2, 6, 27, 96, 205
Thiazides, 33, 119, 132, 134, 210
Thiopentone, 173–175, 180–182, 216
Tranexamic acid, 150, 151, 215
Type 1 diabetes, 118, 119, 124
Type 2 diabetes, 115, 117

V

Vasopressors, 47, 52
Vaughan-Williams classification, 23–25, 209
Volume of distribution, 17, 18, 73, 176, 204
Vomiting reflex, 155

W

Warfarin, 2, 6–8, 17, 26, 41, 63, 66, 88, 96, 97, 99, 119, 147, 148, 150, 152, 156, 158, 159, 214

MIX
Papier aus verantwortungsvollen Quellen
Paper from responsible sources
FSC® C105338

If you have any concerns about our products,
you can contact us on
ProductSafety@springernature.com

In case Publisher is established outside the EU,
the EU authorized representative is:
Springer Nature Customer Service Center GmbH
Europaplatz 3, 69115 Heidelberg, Germany

Printed by Libri Plureos GmbH
in Hamburg, Germany